Meniscus of the Knee - Function, Pathology and Management

Edited by Taiceer Abdulwahab and Karl Almqvist

Published in London, United Kingdom

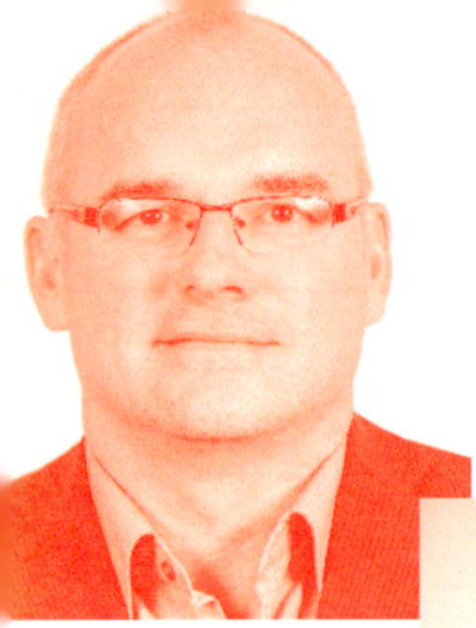
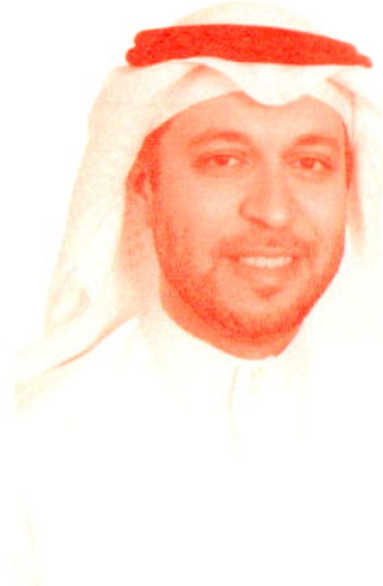
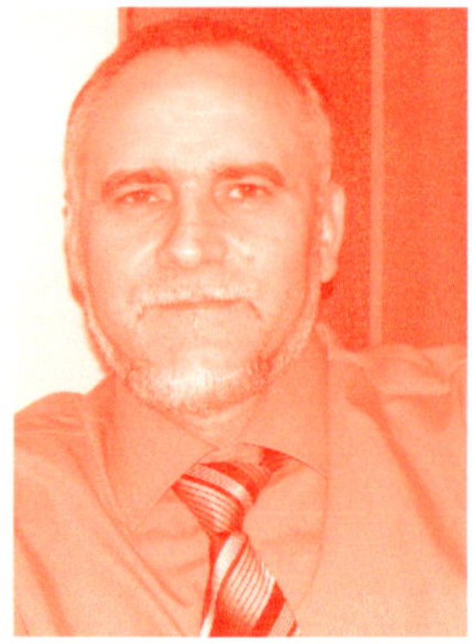
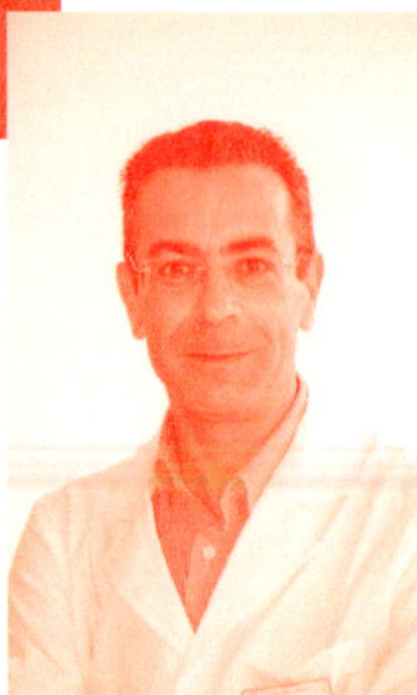
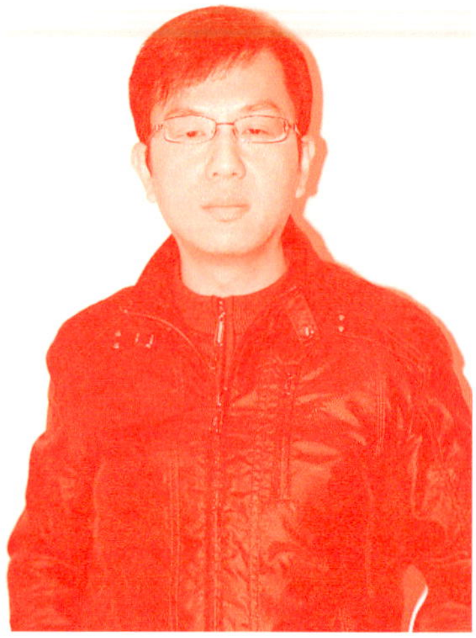
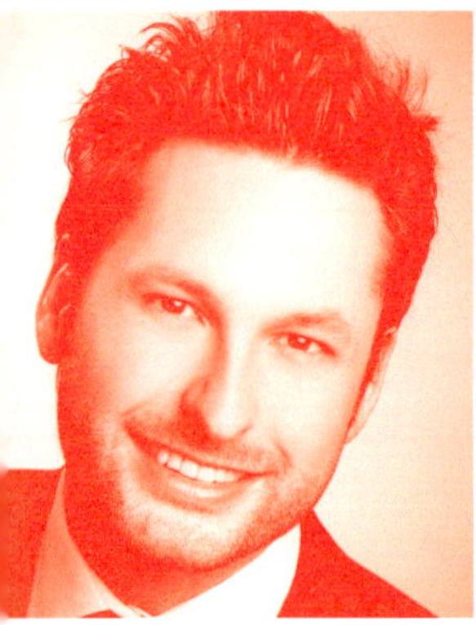
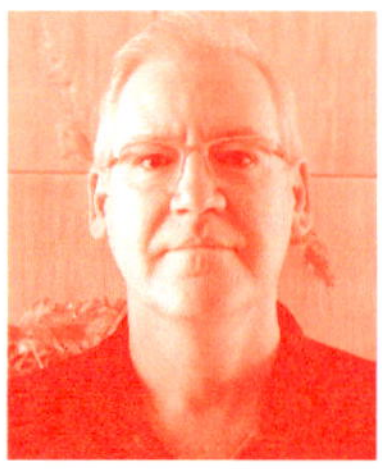

IntechOpen

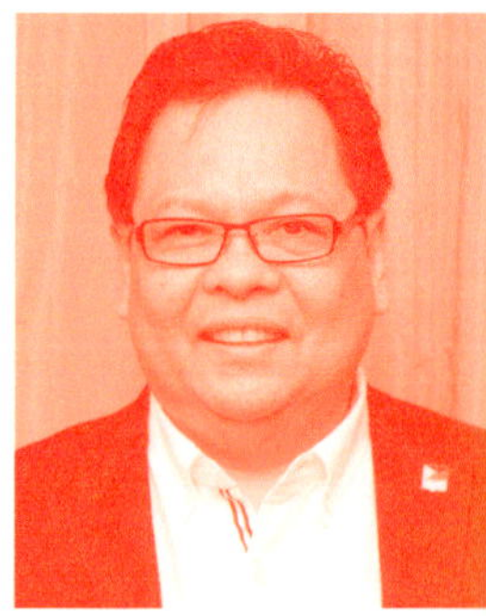
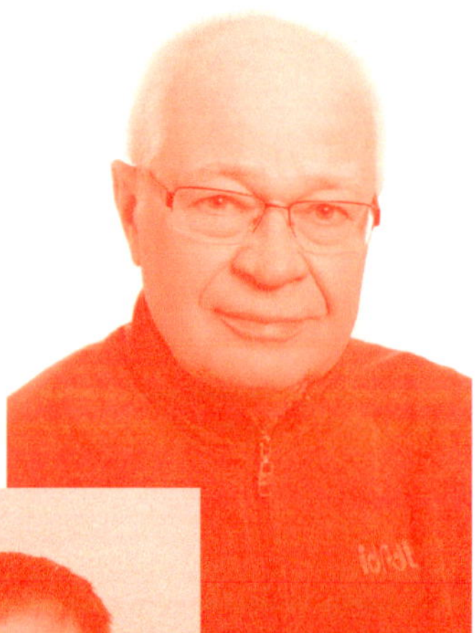
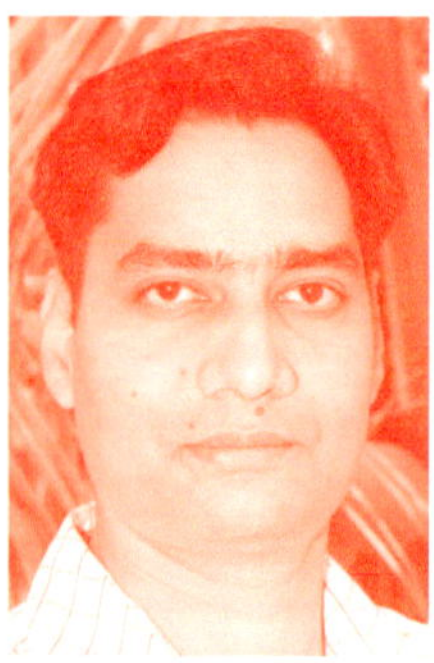
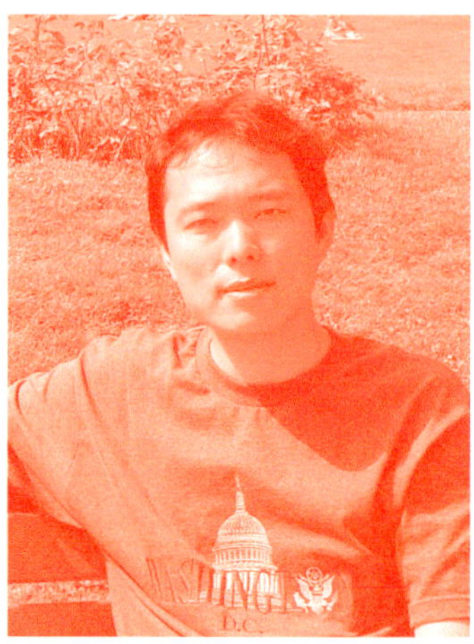
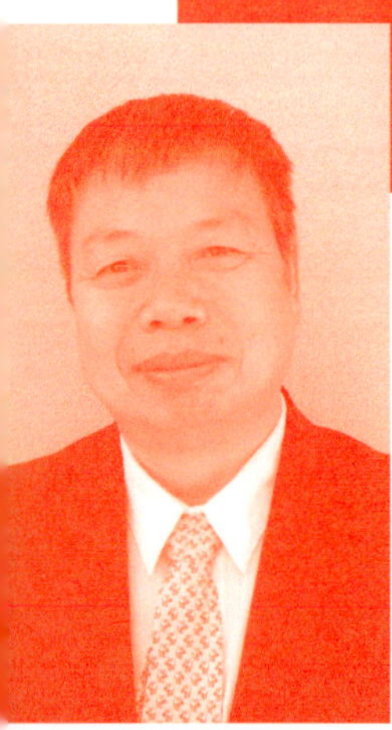
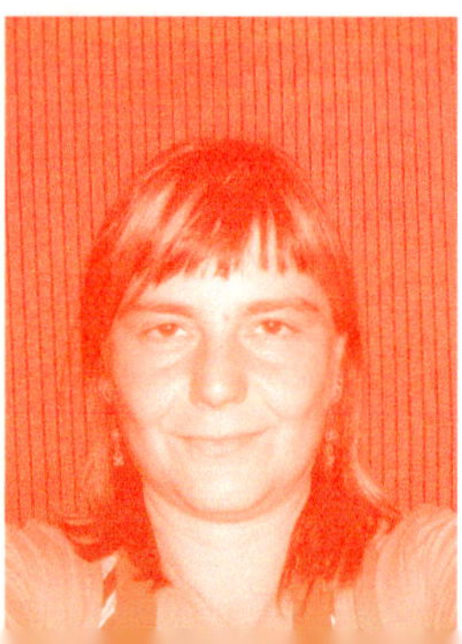

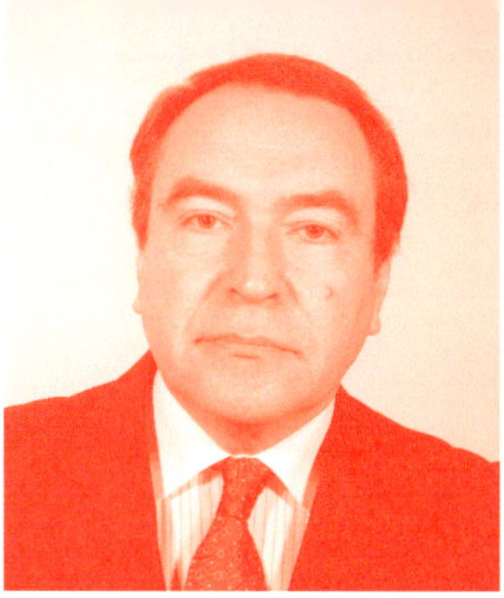
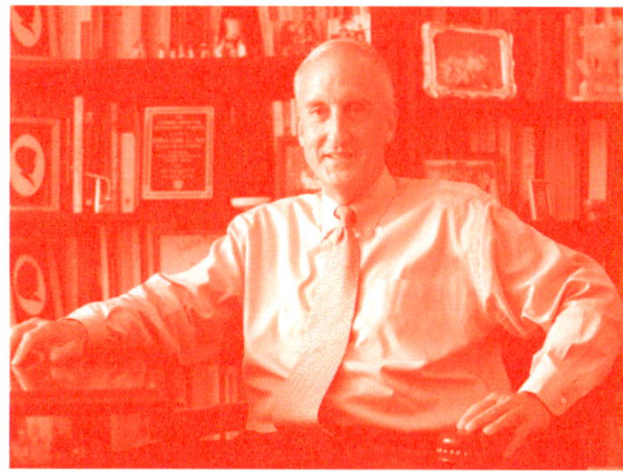
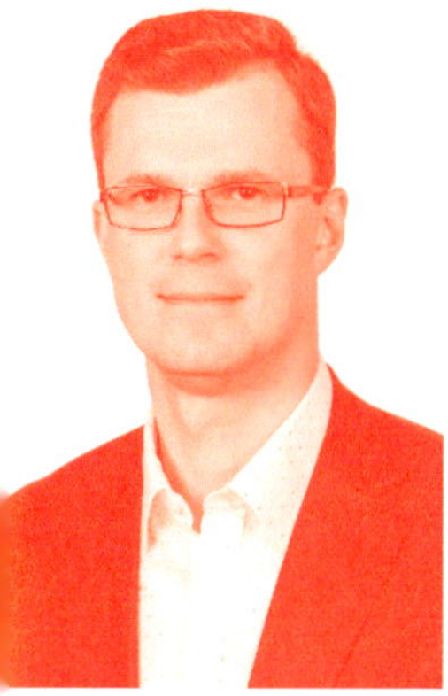
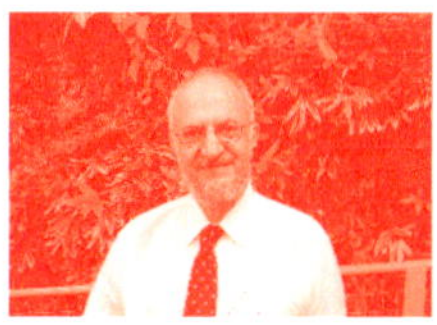
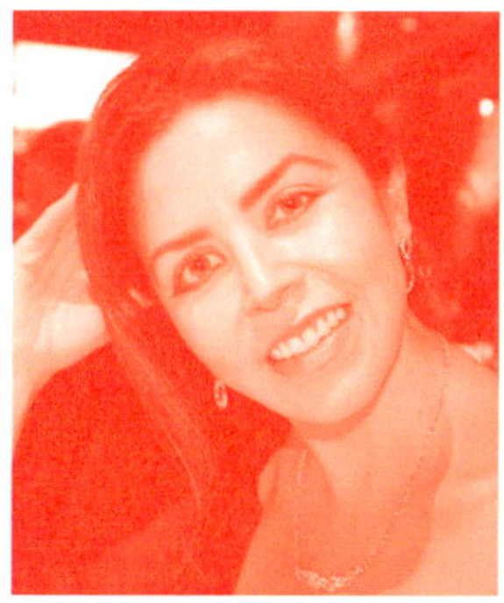

Supporting open minds since 2005

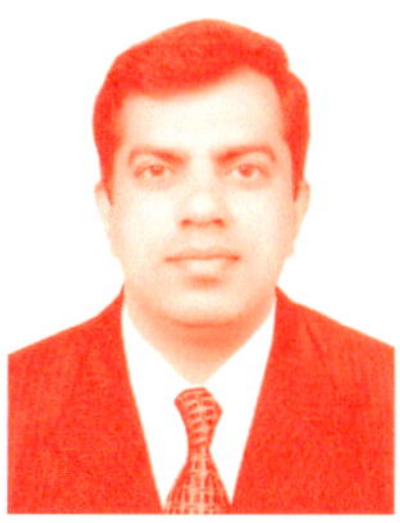
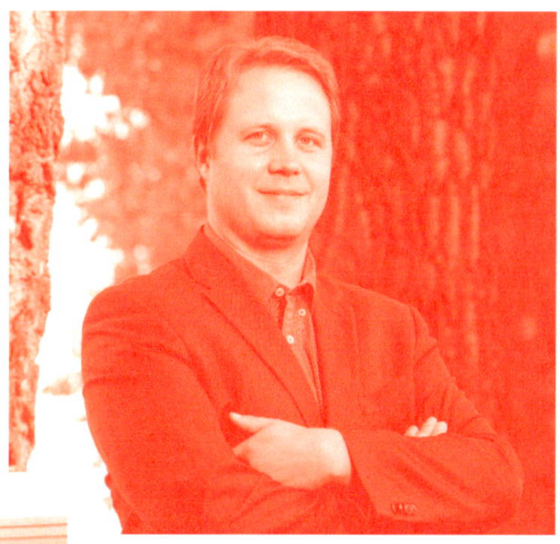
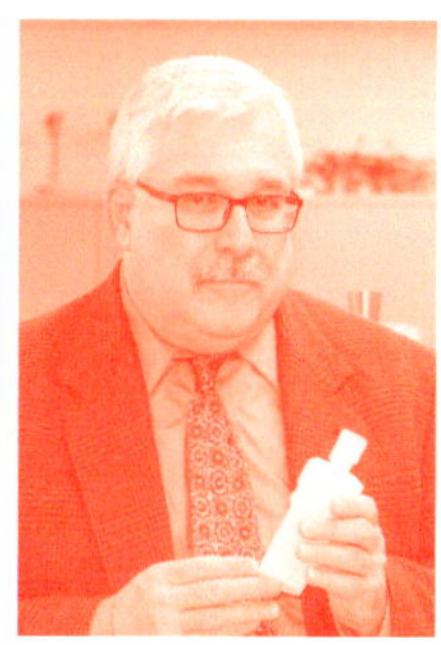
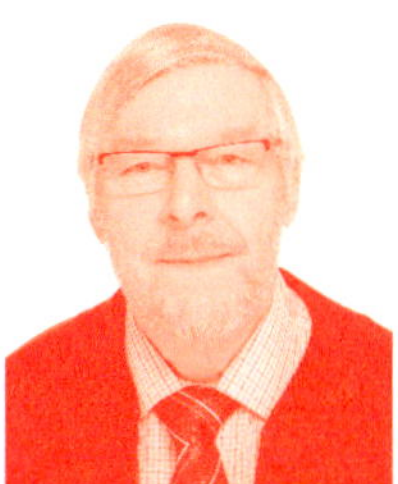
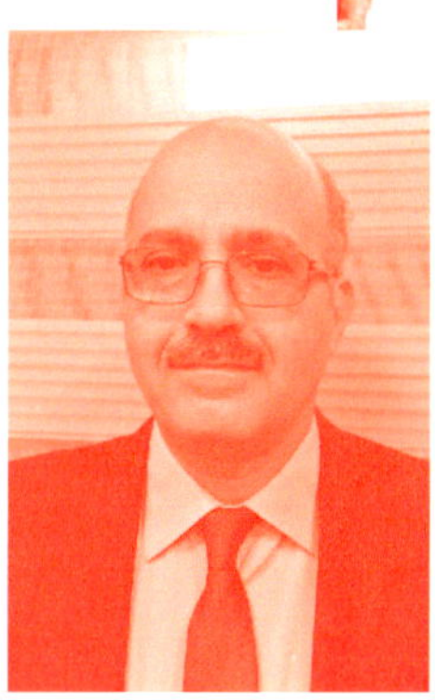
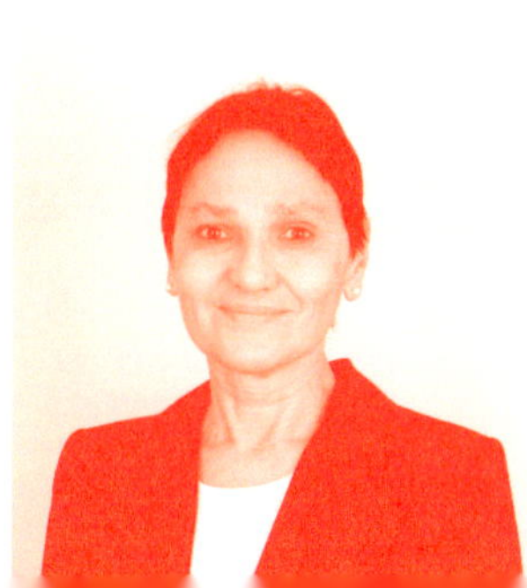
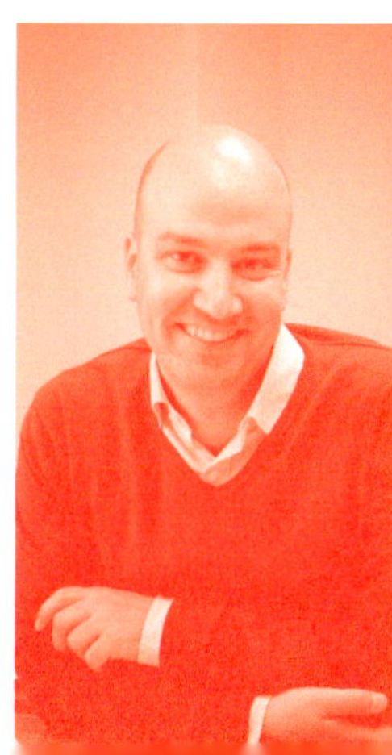

Meniscus of the Knee - Function, Pathology and Management
http://dx.doi.org/10.5772/intechopen.76740
Edited by Taiceer Abdulwahab and Karl Almqvist

Contributors
Vaso Kecojevic, Srdjan Ninkovic, Vladimir Harhaji, James Melrose, Azran Azhim, Najian Ibrahim, Fatihah Yusof, Yaşar Mahsut Dinçel, Abdülkadir Sarı, Burak Günaydın

First published in London, United Kingdom, 2019 by IntechOpen
IntechOpen is the global imprint of INTECHOPEN LIMITED, registered in England and Wales, registration number: 11086078, The Shard, 25th floor, 32 London Bridge Street
London, SE19SG - United Kingdom
Printed in Croatia

British Library Cataloguing-in-Publication Data
A catalogue record for this book is available from the British Library

Additional hard and PDF copies can be obtained from orders@intechopen.com

Meniscus of the Knee - Function, Pathology and Management
Edited by Taiceer Abdulwahab and Karl Almqvist
p. cm.
Print ISBN 978-1-83880-871-6
Online ISBN 978-1-83880-872-3
eBook (PDF) ISBN 978-1-83880-873-0

For EU product safety concerns:
IN TECH d.o.o., Prolaz Marije Krucifikse Kozulić 3, 51000 Rijeka, Croatia, info@intechopen.com or visit our website at intechopen.com.

Meet the editors

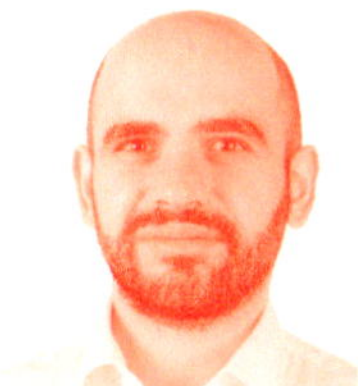

Dr. Taiceer Abdulwahab is an orthopedic surgeon at Mediclinic City Hospital, Dubai, and Clinical Lecturer of Orthopedic Surgery at the College of Medicine, Mohammed Bin Rashid University of Medicine and Health Sciences, Dubai Healthcare City. He holds a Master of Surgery (ChM) degree in Trauma and Orthopedic Surgery from the University of Edinburgh School of Medicine in partnership with the Royal College of Surgeons of Edinburgh, UK. He received his MSc in Trauma and Orthopedic Surgery from Warwick School of Medicine, University of Warwick, UK. Dr. Abdulwahab obtained his primary medical qualification, MB, and ChB from the Bristol School of Medicine, University of Bristol, UK. He has presented at various international conferences, published in peer-reviewed journals, and served as principal investigator in several randomized controlled trials. He is a trauma doctor for the annual Emirates Rugby Sevens. He has a special interest in sports surgery, particularly arthroscopic shoulder and knee surgery.

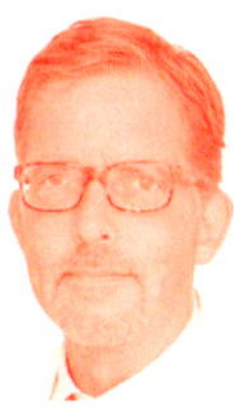

Karl Fredrik Almqvist is an internationally recognized orthopedic surgeon whose main area of interest is knee surgery. His expertise covers the whole range of knee conditions from sports injuries to knee replacement. He trained at the University of Ghent in Belgium and worked at the Ghent University Hospital where he was Head of Clinic, Department of Physical Medicine and Orthopaedic Surgery, prior to moving to Dubai in 2014. He also has considerable teaching experience and is an assistant professor in physiotherapy and orthopedic surgery at Ghent University. Prof. Dr. Almqvist has published extensively and written a number of book chapters. He is a regular speaker at international meetings and is on the editorial board of or is a reviewer for major sports orthopedic journals. He is active in a number of orthopedic organizations, and is the past Chairman of the Sports Committee of the International Society of Arthroscopy, Knee Surgery and Orthopaedic Sports Medicine, as well as the past Chairman of the Cartilage Committee of the European Society of Sports Traumatology, Knee Surgery and Arthroscopy.

Contents

Preface

The principal aim of this book is to provide the arthroscopic orthopaedic surgeon with a clear, concise account of the anatomy, pathology, and conservative and operative surgical techniques in the management of meniscal lesions.

Meniscal lesions are extremely common, and arthroscopic meniscal surgery is one of the most common orthopaedic surgical procedures performed. Therefore the first section of this book ensures an adequate understanding of the anatomy and related pathological process involved in order to provide the reader with a basis for the diagnosis and treatment of meniscal pathology.

The art of meniscal surgery involves many steps, with ever-evolving techniques and implants. It is essential to perform an adequate arthroscopic technique to access all anterior, middle, and posterior thirds of the medial and lateral compartments and the central pivot, as described in the second section of the book.

The final section discusses meniscal preservation techniques, where the aim is to reconstruct a bioengineered meniscus. This is achieved through a combination of scaffolding techniques augmented with biological (extracellular matrix), chemical (acids, enzymes), and physical methods such as sonication decellurisation techniques.

This book has been prepared during a period of widespread debate on, and evolution in, the conservative, surgical, and biological techniques for managing meniscal lesions.

This text will help consolidate the current evidence to enable the development of optimal management plans for meniscal injuries.

Dr. Taiceer Abdulwahab
Orthopaedic Surgeon
Mediclinic City Hospital
Dubai Healthcare City, United Arab Emirates

Clinical Lecturer of Orthopaedic Surgery
College of Medicine
Mohammed Bin Rashid University of Medicine and Health Sciences
Dubai Healthcare City, United Arab Emirates

Karl Almqvist
Professor of Orthopaedic Surgery
Mediclinic City Hospital
Dubai Healthcare City, United Arab Emirates

Section 1

Anatomy of the Meniscus

Chapter 1

Meniscus Tears and Review of the Literature

Abdülkadir Sari, Burak Günaydin and Yaşar Mahsut Dinçel

Abstract

The knee joint is the largest and most complicated joint in the human body. Bone structures, capsules, menisci, and ligaments provide static stability in the knee joint and are responsible for dynamic stabilization of the muscles and tendons. Menisci are fibrocartilage structures that cover two-thirds of the tibial plateau joint surface. The main functions of the meniscus are load sharing and loading of the tibiofemoral joint, shock absorption, helping to feed the cartilage by facilitating dissociation of the joint fluid, and contributing to the joint fit by increasing joint stability and joint contact surface area. Menisci are frequently injured structures. The incidence of acute meniscal tears is 60 per 100,000. It is more common in males. Trauma-related tears are common in patients under 30 years of age, whereas degenerative complex tears increase in patients over 30 years of age. There may not be a significant trauma story, especially in degenerative meniscus tears. They are sports traumas that come to the fore in the etiology of meniscus tears. It is the football that has the greatest risk of creating a meniscus lesion, followed by athletics, American football, and skiing. There is an indication for repair in peripheral ruptures where blood flow is excessive. In the central rupture where blood is not present, the treatment is meniscectomy. In this review, we compiled the diagnosis, etiology, and treatment methods of the meniscal tears.

Keywords: meniscus tears, treatment, sports, trauma, literature, rehabilitation

1. Introduction

The knee is an open joint to frequent injuries in sports activities. Direct impacts, forced movements, or repetitive overloads can cause anatomical damage. Menisci are formed from fibrous cartilage. It has a shock-absorbing feature. The main tasks are providing load transfer, increasing joint surface contact area and joint stability, and contributing to proprioception [1, 2]. A total of 100,000 people per year are found to have meniscus rupture in 60–70 [3]. The most common pathology associated with meniscal tears is anterior cruciate ligament (ACL) ruptures [4].

Today, in addition to professional sportsmen, people participate in sports activities for hobby purposes [5]. Increasing interest in sports with high risk of injury, such as skiing, snowboarding, and mountain biking, has increased the frequency of traumatic meniscal tear [6, 7]. Decision-making process is difficult in professional sportsmen. Approximately 40% of all sports injuries involve the knee joint. Meniscus injuries account for 14.5% of these injuries [6]. The most risky period in terms of age is between the ages of 20 and 29 [6]. Male to female ratio of meniscus proplemia in sports injuries is 2–4/1 [8, 9]. The medial-lateral meniscus injury rate for all age groups was reported as 3/1. However, lateral meniscus tears are more common in young professional athletes [6]. According to the age distribution, the medial meniscus tear is more likely to occur in the athletes who are under 30 years old and laterally in sportsmen over 30 years [10]. In an epidemiological study of National Basketball Association (NBA) basketball players, 87.8% of meniscal tears are isolated, and 12.2% are associated with ligament injuries, often ACL [10]. Acute ACL injuries are more common in lateral meniscus, and chronic ACL injuries are more common in medial meniscus tears [11]. Body mass index (BMI) is specified in professional basketball players as a risk factor. It has been reported that especially above 25, it increases the risk of rupture more in the lateral meniscus [12]. The high physical activity during play was more associated with the lateral meniscus [11]. In an epidemiological study of athletic knee injuries, the distribution of 836 medial meniscus injuries according to sports branches was examined. Soccer was 32.7%, skiing 22.4%, tennis 7.8%, handball 5.4%, and cycling 3.5%. In the distribution of 284 lateral meniscus injuries, 34.5% of football, 19% of skiing, 9.8% of handball, 6.6% of tennis, and 3.5% of cycling sources were stated. In gymnastics and dancers doing lateral, tennis, and jogging, the risk of medial meniscus injuries is greater [6]. Most of the injuries occur during the competition and are thought to be caused by faulty warming or overloading [6]. 10–19 years is the period when lateral meniscus injuries are seen in sportsmen at the second frequency [6]. It is thought that rapid and variable physiology of the age of growth has increased meniscus injuries in this age group [11]. Nowadays, with the understanding of biomechanics and functions of the meniscus, tissue preservation has become the mainstay of treatment [7]. Exposure to high physical activity levels and relatively early age causes injury to the athletes in terms of degenerative arthrosis [7].

The diagnosis of symptomatic meniscus rupture can be made during the anatomy of the patient. The common complaints of patients are pain during hanging and flexion, which starts after the knee swelling or excessive flexion. On physical examination, joint tenderness, McMurray test, and Apley test were described as the most commonly used tests [8]. Magnetic resonance imaging (MRI) can diagnose approximately 95% of cases. Because non-symptomatic individuals can also detect meniscal tears with MRI, treatment decisions should be made by combining them with the clinical findings of the patient, not just the MRI outcome [13]. Many features should be taken into account when deciding on surgical treatment of meniscus tears. Among the factors that are effective in deciding on surgical technique for menisci are patient complaints, age, rupture size, and additional pathologies associated with morphology [14].

Total meniscectomy has been used extensively in the pre-arthroscopic era and has caused many athletes to lose their sporting life [15]. It has been shown that partial meniscectomy causes irreversible damage to joint cartilage in the long term [16]. Since the 1980s, the development of arthroscopic techniques and the ability to repair the menstrual blood, and thus the healing possibilities, have led to the repair of suitable tears. Longitudinal tears, usually in the peripheral 25% area, are suitable for repairs in young and sporty people. With the understanding that menisci are indispensable for knee health today, indications for repair especially in lateral meniscus tears have been expanded.

In the beginning, conventional sewing techniques have been described as repairs from the inside to the outside and from the outside [17]. With a variety of meniscal fixators (meniscus fixation materials), the possibility of vascular nerve injury with complete internal repair has been reduced, and operation times have been shortened [18].

In comparison with biomechanical stitches, conventional stitches have shown remarkably superior durability than meniscal fixators in many studies [19].

When performing arthroscopic surgery, care should first be taken to protect the meniscus tissue. Accompanying lesions should be evaluated carefully, especially with frequent ACL problems. All problems should be solved together by following a holistic approach in treatment. These injuries cause serious morbidity in the short term when not properly treated. In the long term, it may also lead to degenerative changes in the knee joint resulting in osteoarthritis.

Therefore, the treatment of meniscus injuries is very important. Today, it is understood that meniscus is protected as much as possible. Current treatment methods are being implemented and developed on the basis of this principle [20].

In this article, we aim to present the latest developments in diagnosis, treatment, and follow-up of meniscus injuries in the light of the literature.

2. Meniscus tear

Meniscus tears are the result of traumatic, degenerative, or congenital pathologies. Loads exceeding the normal endurance limit may result in a tear. In degenerative menisci, ruptures may also occur at normal loads. Traumatic tears usually occur in active people, aged between 10 and 40 years [10]. Degenerative tears are generally over 40 years of age. Such tears are often associated with other degenerative changes in the cartilage and bone tissues of the knee.

3. Management of treatment

Accelerating degenerative changes in the meniscus-deficient knees and the menisci played a key role in the functioning of the meniscus leading us to focus on the protection of the meniscus. In early 1948, Fairbank showed that total meniscectomy accelerated the radiological change in the knee [21]. This was changed by partial meniscectomy [22].

There is no randomized controlled trial showing that arthroscopic meniscus repair has a long-term benefit for joint protection. However, good results to date suggest that this may reduce the incidence of early degenerative changes [23].

According to De Haven, all meniscus tears would not cause clinical symptoms [24]. It has been shown that the tibial asymptomatic meniscus tears, which are intact and have biomechanical function, can recover spontaneously.

The results of not treating meniscus tears are not very clear. Experimental animal studies have shown that meniscal tears may result in chondropathy and osteoarthritis [25, 26].

Clinical studies could not explain whether meniscal injury or articular cartilage damage developed first [27]. A recent study by Christoforakis evaluated 497 consecutive knee arthroscopies in patients with meniscal tear [28]. These complex and horizontal tears were found to be statistically increased in outerbridge [29] grade III or IV joint cartilage damage. Moreover, complex and horizontal tears had excessive joint damage compared to other types of tears. Nevertheless, the result does not answer which of the meniscus tears or articular degeneration occurred first.

The general approach is to actively tear the young patients with clinical and radiological examinations including X-ray and MRI. If there is a tear or is very suspicious, arthroscopy and meniscus protection surgery are recommended.

Non-operative treatment option is used in patients with suspected degenerative tears. The debridement of the degenerated meniscus is well documented that it cannot always result in long-term relief [30].

3.1 Non-operative treatment

Small peripheral tears in young patients can be treated without surgery. The difficulty is to decide whether the tear is stable or not. Weiss et al. retrospectively reviewed 3612 arthroscopic procedures for meniscus lesions [31]. They found 80 (2.2%) meniscus tears which were considered stable. They were not treated. Six patients presented for arthroscopy again due to meniscus symptoms. The authors suggest that stable vertical peripheral tears have a high healing potential [31].

Physiotherapy has been shown to be beneficial to patients with degenerative meniscus tears. In a recent published randomized control study, patients who underwent surgical debridement with physiotherapy showed no better results than those who received only physiotherapy [32].

Some patients with degenerative meniscal tears recover after a single corticosteroid injection into the knee. Corticosteroids are the first-line treatment for degenerative meniscus in the absence of locking symptoms.

Because of the high functional expectations and the need for early return to sports, it is still preferred in selected cases [33].

In the red-red zone, stable, incomplete longitudinal tears with a size below 1 cm may be suitable for conservative treatment [7]. Bucket handle, radial, parrot beak, oblique tears, and degenerative and complex tears are not suitable for conservative methods [34]. Conservative treatment can be used as a temporary treatment method in athletes, who are frequently asymptomatic in the season [33].

Selection should be made when deciding on conservative treatment. Abnormal stresses should be avoided in the early period of rupture. The development of cartilage lesions after aggressive rehabilitation of a young professional athlete with lateral meniscus radial rupture to return to early sports shows that this treatment is not innocent [35]. It should be kept in mind that meniscus tears, which cannot be repaired, may cause cartilage lesions due to mechanical problems that occur even if they are not symptomatic in athletes. Surgical treatment should be prioritized especially in athletes [5].

3.2 Operative management

3.2.1 Total meniscectomy

With the development of arthroscopic techniques and understanding of biomechanics, the importance of meniscus has increased. Treatment led to a shift toward the protection of the meniscus tissue. Total meniscectomy treatment is rarely practiced today.

3.2.2 Open repair

It was one of the first ways to repair meniscus tears [36]. It is now used to fix the meniscus as part of the management of tibial plateau fractures.

3.2.3 Arthroscopic repair

The high expectations and career concerns of the athletes have made the meniscus repairs even more important. Red-red zone often provides successful repairs due to the potential for cannulation. Discussions on repairs to the red-white zone are still ongoing. In a study, midterm and long-term acceptable results after repair of red-white zone tears of 22 athletes are promising [37].

When deciding on the repair of meniscus in professional athletes, it is necessary to take into account the possibility of the meniscus recovery and to target 90% success. Considering the possible risks, the athletes should be careful to repair the tears in the red-white zone. White-white zone is considered to be the indication of repair today. But athletes should not consider arthroscopic repair [5].

Meniscus tear is present in 60% of ACL-ruptured patients [38]. When the ligament is not repaired, the meniscus is becoming more complicated as it is not healed [39]. For this reason, repairs should be done in the early period and in the same session.

Although it is accepted that there is an improvement in the repair area in about 6–8 weeks, the process actually lasts longer, and the athletes cannot return to competitive activities before 3 months [7]. As stated by Forriol's study, the improvement in the repaired meniscus depends on two basic elements. The first one is the extrinsic blood circulation, and the other is the ability to repair synovial fluid and fibrocartilage intrinsically [40]. Histological studies after meniscus repair are based on animal experiments and cannot be fully adapted to human meniscus repair process [41]. Therefore, the relationship between healing in tissue and return to movement is mostly based on clinical observations.

The success rates after repair vary. Pujol et al. reported success rates between 5 and 43% of meniscus repair in basketball players [42]. According to Stein et al. in the 8-year follow-up, the rate of return to pre-traumatic activity in the group undergoing athletes was found to be 96.2%, and in the meniscectomy group, it was 50% [43]. Paxton et al. found failure after meniscectomy was 3.7% and in repair group 20.7% [44]. In this article, better long-term clinical results have been reported in meniscus repairs despite high reoperation rates [44].

It is reported that repair is better characterized by better functional scores and lower failure rates in the current meta-analysis of meniscectomy and repair [45]. Reoperation depends not only on the technique but on the skill of the orthopedist, the tear itself, the age of the athlete, the level of activity, and the rehabilitation program applied [44]. In a study evaluating the results of repair in athletes, failure in the medial meniscus was reported as 36.4%, and failure in the lateral meniscus was reported to be 5.6%.

Reoperation rates are high in medial meniscus repairs. This is due to the less mobility of the medial meniscus and to the greater load on the medial compartment [46]. Late repair of medial tears has also been implicated as the cause of this failure [47].

Forty-two elite athletes and meniscus repair agressively recommend the study, after the repair reported 24% failure. Of the cases, 67% had medial meniscus, and 33% had lateral meniscus tears and a mean follow-up of 8.5 years [47].

The success of repair in the complete radial tears of the lateral meniscus is low [48]. However, in the studies of Haklar et al., successful results are obtained in approximately half of the patients, and return to sports is provided [48]. Nevertheless, these patients should be shared with the athlete who may be a candidate for meniscus transplant in the future.

The surgeon must also make efforts to repair the medial or lateral meniscus radial root tears in athletes. If the circumferential fibers are completely ruptured when the repair is not performed, the meniscus becomes functional. Therefore, primary repair of complete radial tears should be the first aim, especially in young athletes.

Radial tears in the posterior meniscus posterior are more promising because of the region's blood supply [49].

Failure to achieve successful results with today's repair techniques leads to new searches. The success of repair in meniscus tears combined with ACL reconstruction is thought to be the effect of growth factors and multipotent cells from the bone marrow [50]. Similarly, synovial abrasion, trephination, mechanical stimulation, fibrin clot, or platelet-rich plasma (PRP) applications are always aimed for the same purpose [51].

The growth factors released after mechanical stimulation and trephination contribute positively to meniscus healing. Ochi et al. showed that the mediators increased to the highest level in the joint after 14 days of mechanical stimulation [52].

Trephination can be used successfully in the complete tears of the lateral meniscus posterior or in complete longitudinal tears less than 1 cm. Successful results of vertical, peripheral, and non-degenerative tears in trephination are seen in the literature [53].

In a recent study on the effect of PRP on meniscus repairs, no significant difference was found in functional scores [51]. Rights et al. used microfracture to create an effect similar to ACL reconstruction, and this would also contribute positively to recovery in the repair area of multipotent cells.

Studies have shown that smoking has a negative effect on the results of meniscus repair [54].

For successful results, it is important to remember the importance of combining vertical mattress sutures from the inside to the outside as far as possible, with the microfracture method [54].

The presence of opposing views in the literature shows that there is still no consensus on rehabilitation and return to sports after repair [55]. In the conservative approach, the return to sports takes a long period such as 3–6 months, while the aggressive approach is as short as 10 weeks [56]. While limited conservative rehabilitation is recommended initially until the meniscus is healed [57], recent biomechanical studies report that early burden is not inconvenient [58]. Even in animal experiments, it has been shown that blood flow to the repair site increases with mobilization [59].

In a randomized controlled trial by Lind et al., the functional scores with MRI and arthroscopy are evaluated. The rate of failure was found to be 28% in the limited rehabilitation group and 36% in the nonrestricted rehabilitation group [60].

As a result, we can say that the trend toward accelerated rehabilitation in the current studies is promising. In practice, the location of the tear, its size, the quality of the meniscus, and the stability of the repair affect the rehabilitation to be applied to the athlete [5]. Neuromuscular control is very important in current rehabilitation [56]. The individual needs and sports-specific approaches of the athlete should not be ignored in rehabilitation [61].

Meniscal tears in young athletes have great challenges for orthopedists. High activity-level, long career expectancy requires all conditions to be repaired [46]. The high potential of recovery according to adults is an important advantage [11].

Athletes may be asked to be guided by the orthopedist athlete or club when planning treatment. Often, the athlete's desire to return to sports early can create pressure on the physician. The rehabilitation process following the treatment of accompanying ligamentous injuries gives the physician the time required for recovery after meniscus repair [62]. However, the expectation of early sports return to isolated meniscus tears may force the physician to perform meniscectomy. Taking into account the expectations of the athlete and the situation in which he/she is not affected from the orthopedic pressures, it is to make the right decision to give priority to anatomical and functional meniscus repair.

3.2.4 Meniscal rasping

Meniscal rasping is used to clean the torn edges of the meniscus to stimulate bleeding. It is indicated in patients with stable, longitudinal tears in the vascular region of the meniscus. In the case of unstable knee or avascular region ruptures, this treatment is not appropriate.

3.2.5 Meniscal suturing

Red-red zone or red-white zone tears can be repaired. Traditionally, longitudinal tears are most suitable for suturing and healing. The most important condition for a good recovery is a stable knee. Repair of meniscus in unstable knees results in failure of treatment.

However, a stable knee with normal kinematics does not apply unnecessary shear force on the meniscus repair. Recently, positive results have been obtained regarding the repair of full-thickness radial tears [59]. The results of the repair were not reported in randomized controlled trials. However, case reports seem to be positive. Repairs in the avascular region are at risk of failure. Meniscus repair, with ACL reconstruction, showed better recovery rates than ACL stable knees [63].

3.2.6 Meniscal suturing techniques

Various techniques for the repair of meniscus have been described.

3.2.6.1 Outside-in meniscal suturing techniques

It was the first arthroscopic node technique. It is now the least used method. Suitable for tears in the middle and anterior 1/3 section of the meniscus. Posterior 1/3 cut is not possible with this technique.

The most important advantages of the outside-in repair method are that it is very easy to reach the anterior 1/3 region ruptures which are difficult to reach by other methods and it does not require additional posteromedial or posterolateral cuts to protect the vascular nerve pack. The most important disadvantage of this method is the difficulty in reaching tears extending to the posterior 1/3.

3.2.6.2 Inside-out meniscal suturing techniques

Single- or double-lumen, special-inclined cannula through the needles passed through the repair. It can be applied to tears in every region, but it is more suitable for tears in the rear and middle 1/3 section. With this method, which is accepted as the gold standard in meniscus repair, the desired number and type of stitches can be placed easily in each region of the meniscus.

The most important disadvantage of the method is the need for a second incision in the posteromedial or posterolateral to prevent the needles from the capsule from causing vascular nerve injury, requiring an experienced assistant and special instrumentation.

The repair of tears near the posterior insertion of the meniscus is difficult and dangerous with the inside-out technique. In this type of tear, Morgan described the whole technique of sewing inside [64].

4. Meniscus fixators

Implants called “meniscus fixators” have been developed due to the difficulties of sewing techniques, in some cases requiring additional incisions and vascular nerve complications. These implants manufactured as arrow, hook, anchor, screw, or staple are biodegradable or permanent.

The most important advantage of the fixators is that they are technically very easy. In addition, there are advantages such as very low vascular nerve complications, no need for additional incisions, meniscus tears in hard-to-reach areas, "all-in-one" repair, no assistant, and no need for arthroscopic nodes. Generally, there is no problem in the visualization of the lateral compartment. Medial repair on very narrow knees can be difficult [65].

However, the fixators have serious disadvantages. The mechanical forces are half or one-third of the vertical stitch [66].

Another problem with meniscus fixators is the risk of rigid implants to damage the articular cartilage [19]. This problem arises especially in puffy head implants, which are not fully embedded in the meniscus body.

5. Methods for improving the healing

Methods for improving healing in tears extending to the nonvascular area have been described. Some authors recommend applying one or more of these methods in all isolated tears, regardless of the area in which they are located. These methods are described below.

5.1 Fibrin clot technique

When the patient's venous blood is mixed with a glass baguette, the paste-shaped clot is placed between the torn lips. Since Arnoczky showed the chemotactic and mitogenic factors involved in these dogs and showed that this clot had a positive effect on healing, this technique was also introduced in humans [67].

5.2 Trephination technique

This method is based on the principle of opening radial tunnels in the meniscus body so that the peripheral vascular structures reach the avascular region. Zhang et al. showed that the trephination combined with the suture was more effective than the suture alone in avascular tears in the goat meniscus [68, 69].

5.3 Synovial abrasion

It is based on the principle of a hemorrhage and infusion responses as a result of filing the synovial tissue around the rupture with the help of a curette and contributing to the healing process [70].

5.4 Synovial flap transfer

It was shown that a better repair tissue was formed in the animal experiments with the interposition of a vascular tissue, a pedicled flap, in the tear area of the synovium [71]. However, this technique has not been widely used.

5.5 Texture adhesives

An ideal tissue adhesive should include the following: tissue compatibility, biodegradable, good connect, minimal tissue reaction, and affordable [72].

Tissue adhesives currently used in clinical practice are limited because they contain all of these features.

5.6 Growth factors in meniscus repair

It is known that fibrin clots placed in meniscus tears increase the healing potential of these lesions. It has been shown that meniscal fibrochondrocytes have the ability to make matrix and cell proliferation when they are associated with mitogenic and chemotactic factors in wound hematoma [73]. In fibrochondrocyte cell culture, platelet-derived growth factor (PDGF) has been shown to stimulate proliferation of these cells [74].

Researchers showed that PDGF alone could not initiate meniscus repair in the central region of the meniscus [74].

The effect of endothelial cell growth factor (ECGF) on the healing potential of meniscal injuries was investigated. It has been said that there is not much effect [72].

6. Rehabilitation in patients with meniscus repair

The discussion in the literature is on rehabilitation protocols that should be applied after isolated meniscus repair [75]. There is no consensus on knee movement, weight-bearing, knee pad use, and return to sports. In more conservative protocols, there are 4–6 weeks of partial load, knee movements gradually increased in knee pad control, and 6 months of deep crouching and sports ban. In contrast, aggressive protocols recommend immediate burdening, unlimited knee movement, and return to sports when muscle strength is acquired, as long as the patient can tolerate it.

In 95 patients with aggressive and conservative protocols, there was no difference in failure rates [75]. This study yields full knee movement width and allows for return to sports when pain and effusion are lost. Since the only factor affecting the success of the repair is not rehabilitation, the results of various series are difficult to compare. The generally accepted opinion is that rehabilitation using only meniscus fixators is a little more conservative.

7. Scaffolds

Scaffolds can be used as salvage interventions in meniscus ruptures with irreparable meniscus tears and athletes with segmental meniscectomy [7]. The porous and absorbable structure should provide a meniscus-like tissue formation, while the biomechanical strength of the joint should be adequate.

In a European-centered study, 52 partial meniscectomy patients underwent polyurethane scaffold. In the third month, 81.4% of the patients underwent MRI. In the 12th month of the arthroscopic evaluation, in 97.7% of the cases, scaffold integration was detected with real meniscus tissue [76]. Zaffagnini et al. 43 patients with lateral menisectomy applied scaffold. At the sixth postoperative month, they showed functional improvement. At the 12th month, the knee swelling and fatigue decreased to the optimal level. At the 24-month follow-up, 58% of the cases had reached the pre-injury activity level, and 95% of the patients had patient satisfaction [77].

However, it is recommended not to give a full load for 6–8 weeks after meniscus scaffold applications. This causes muscle atrophy especially in athletes and is inadequate to prevent rehabilitation muscle atrophy [78].

Nowadays, cell scaffolds have been introduced. The benefit of cell-free scaffolds was questioned [40]. The factors affecting the success of the procedure were indicated as chronicity of the injury, body mass index, and other accompanying knee problems [48]. Long-term studies on the results of scaffold applications, especially in athletes, are needed.

8. Meniscus transplantation

Meniscus transplantation has been proposed to prevent the development of arthrosis in young patients whose meniscus is completely removed, without axial impairment and arthritic changes. The structures used for meniscus replacement in experimental and clinical studies are as follows: autografts, allografts, xenografts, synthetic polymer implants, carbon fiber and polyurethane implants [79].

It is doubtful that structures used as meniscus transplant may prevent the development of arthritis in the knee in the long term [79].

8.1 Allograft transplantation

Subtotal or total meniscectomy after the functional deficiency and pain is applied in athletes [80]. After close meniscectomy, especially under the influence of abnormal load distribution in the lateral compartment, chondral lesions develop in the early period. The rehabilitation of an athlete who develops a chondral lesion is more difficult, and in the late period, arthrosis develops frequently [81]. For success in transplantation, it is important that the articular cartilage surface is smooth, stable, and normal or that BMI is below 30. In a recent meta-analysis, good and excellent results were reported in 84% of cases after transplantation.

Again in a recent study, posttransplantation in 12 professional footballers was performed in 92% of the cases. At the 36th month, 75% of the cases were reported to continue their professional sports lives [59].

Studies and discussions on transplantation still continue, with short-term to midterm results being positive [82]. There is a rare risk of infection [83]. The delay in returning to sports due to the long healing process is the biggest obstacle to the technique. Currently, randomized controlled long-term studies are needed [34].

It should be kept in mind that this intervention can be applied after the professionalism of the athletes who have undergone meniscectomy in their careers and who are symptomatic or postponed transplantation in their careers.

9. Conclusion

Meniscus injuries constitute a large part of the studies performed by orthopedist surgeons. The current management has progressed toward the meniscus protection. Although there has been a lot of progress in meniscus transplantation, this has still not become a routine procedure.

Young athletes need to make more efforts to protect the meniscus, while long-term treatments in a professional athlete may be postponed at the end of their career. Radial tears of the lateral meniscus corpus and anterior junction are quite important in athletes. They need to be treated early. In the case of complete radial tears, the rate of recovery after repair should be tried, but it should be noted that these patients may be transplant candidates in the later period.

Author details

Abdülkadir Sari, Burak Günaydin and Yaşar Mahsut Dinçel*
Department of Orthopedics and Traumatology, Faculty of Medicine, Namık Kemal University, Tekirdag, Turkey

*Address all correspondence to: ymd61@hotmail.com

References

[1] Kılıç B. Six year follow-up after arthroscopic meniscectomy. Advances in Environmental Biology. 2015;**9**(2):50-53

[2] Indelli PF, Szivek JA, Schnepp AS, Grana AW. Load bearing at the meniscofemoral joint. The Duke Orthopaedic Journal. 2010-2011;**1**(1):39-43

[3] Alturfan AK, Kılıçoğlu Ö, Gür E. Menisküs sorunları. Türkiye Klinikleri Ortopedi ve Travmatoloji Dergisi. 2006;**39**:23-30

[4] Kilcoyne KG, Dickens JF, Haniuk E, Cameron KL, Owens BD. Epidemiology of meniscal injury associated with ACL tears in young athletes. Orthopedics. 2012;**35**(3):208-212

[5] Meniscus. TUSYAD. Educational Book Series. Chapter 21. 2016. pp. 57-59

[6] Majewski M, Susanne H, Klaus S. Epidemiology of athletic knee injuries: A 10-year study. The Knee. 2006;**13**(3):184-188

[7] Zedde P, Mela F, Del Prete F, Masia F, Manunta AF. Joints. 2015;**2**(4):192-196. eCollection Oct–Dec 2014

[8] Greis PE, Bardana DD, Holmstrom MC, Burks RT. Meniscal injury: I. Basic science and evaluation. The Journal of the American Academy of Orthopaedic Surgeons. 2002;**10**(3):168-117

[9] Baker BE, Peckham AC, Pupparo F, Sanborn JC. Review of meniscal injury and associated sports. The American Journal of Sports Medicine. 1985;**13**(1):1-4

[10] Yeh PC, Starkey C, Lombardo S, Vitti G, Kharrazi FD. Epidemiology of isolated meniscal injury and its effect on performance in athletes from the National Basketball Association. The American Journal of Sports Medicine. 2012;**40**(3):589-594

[11] Popkin CA, Murnaghan ML. Knee injuries in the growing athlete. Orthopaedics and Traumatology. 2012;**26**(1):12-19

[12] Poulsen MR, Johnson DL. Meniscal injuries in the young, athletically active patient. The Physician and Sportsmedicine. 2011;**39**(1):123-130

[13] LaPrade RF, Burnett QM II, Veenstra MA, Hodgman CG. The prevalence of abnormal magnetic resonance imaging findings in asymptomatic knees: With correlation of magnetic resonance imaging to arthroscopic findings in symptomatic knees. The American Journal of Sports Medicine. 1994;**22**:739-745

[14] Metcalf RW, Burks RT, Metcalf MS, McGinty JB. Arthroscopic meniscectomy. In: McGinty JB, Caspari RB, Jackson RW, Poehling GG, editors. Operative Arthroscopy. 2nd ed. Philadelphia, PA: Lippincott-Raven; 1996. pp. 263-297

[15] Bonneux I, Vandekerckhove B. Arthroscopic partial lateral meniscectomy long-term results in athletes. Acta Orthopaedica Belgica. 2002;**68**:356-361

[16] Jaureguito JW, Elliot JS, Lietner T, Dixon LB, Reider B. The effects of arthroscopic partial lateral meniscectomy in an otherwise normal knee: A retrospective review of functional, clinical, and radiographic results. Arthroscopy. 1995;**11**(1):29-36

[17] Cannon WD Jr, Morgan CD. Meniscal repair: Arthroscopic repair techniques. Instructional Course Lectures. 1994;**43**:77-96

[18] Lozano J, Ma CB, Cannon WD. All inside meniscus repair. Clinical

Orthopaedics and Related Research. 2006;**455**:134-141

[19] Barber FA, Herbert MA. Meniscal repair devices. Arthroscopy. 2000;**16**(6):613-618

[20] Fox AJ, Bedi A, Rodeo SA. The basic science of human knee menisci: Structure, composition, and function. Sports Health. 2012;**4**(4):340-351

[21] Fairbank TJ. Knee joint changes after meniscectomy. The Journal of Bone and Joint Surgery. American Volume. 1948;**30B**(4):664-670

[22] Hulet CH, Locker BG, Schiltz D, Texier A, Tallier E, Vielpeau CH. Arthroscopic medial meniscectomy on stable knees. Journal of Bone and Joint Surgery. British Volume (London). 2001;**83**(1):29-32

[23] Sohn DH, Moorman CT. Meniscal debridement: Current concepts. The Journal of Knee Surgery. 2008;**21**(2):145-153

[24] De Haven KE. Decision-making factors in the treatment of meniscus lesions. Clinical Orthopaedics. 1990;**252**:49-54

[25] Appleyard RC, Burkhardt D, Ghosh P, Read R, Cake M, Swain MV, et al. Topographical analysis of the structural, biochemical and dynamic biomechanical properties of cartilage in an ovine model of osteoarthritis. Osteoarthritis and Cartilage. 2003;**11**(1):65-77

[26] Janusz MJ, Bendele AM, Brown KK, Taiwo YO, Hsieh L, Heitmeyer SA. Induction of osteoarthritis in the rat by surgical tear of the meniscus: Inhibition of joint damage by a matrix metalloproteinase inhibitor. Osteoarthritis and Cartilage. 2002;**10**(10):785-791

[27] Fahmy NR, Williams EA, Noble J. Meniscal pathology and osteoarthritis of the knee. Journal of Bone and Joint Surgery. British Volume (London). 1983;**65**(1):24-28

[28] Christoforakis J, Pradhan R, Sanchez-Ballester J, Hunt N, Strachan RK. Is there an association between articular cartilage changes and degenerative meniscus tears? Arthroscopy. 2005;**21**(11):1366-1369

[29] Outerbridge RE. The etiology of chondromalacia patellae. Journal of Bone and Joint Surgery. British Volume (London). 1961;**43-B**:752-757

[30] Matsusue Y, Thomson NL. Arthroscopic partial medial meniscectomy in patients over 40 years old: A 5- to 11 year follow-up study. Arthroscopy. 1996;**12**(1):39-44

[31] Weiss CB, Lundberg M, Hamberg P, DeHaven KE, Gillquist J. Non-operative treatment of meniscal tears. The Journal of Bone and Joint Surgery. American Volume. 1989;**71**(6):811-822

[32] Herrlin S, Hallander M, Wange P, Weidenhielm L, Werner S. Arthroscopic or conservative treatment of degenerative medial meniscal tears: A prospective randomised trial. Knee Surgery, Sports Traumatology, Arthroscopy. 2007;**15**(4):393-401

[33] Bizzini M, Gorelick M, Drobny T. Lateral meniscus repair in a professional ice hockey goaltender: A case report with a 5-year follow-up. The Journal of Orthopaedic and Sports Physical Therapy. 2006;**36**(2):89-100

[34] Giuliani JR, Burns TC, Svoboda SJ, Cameron KL, Owens BD. Treatment of meniscal injuries in young athletes. The Journal of Knee Surgery. 2011;**24**(2):93-100

[35] Thaunat M, Archbold P, Conteduca J, Chatellard R, Sonnery-Cottet B. Rapid chondrolysis following an unoperated lateral meniscus tear in a young

professional rugby player. Orthopaedics & Traumatology, Surgery & Research. 2014;**100**(4):445-448

[36] De Haven KE, Sebastianelli WJ. Open meniscus repair. Indications, technique, and results. Clinics in Sports Medicine. 1990;**9**(3):577-587

[37] Noyes FR, Chen RC, Barber-Westin SD, Potter HG. Greater than 10-year results of red-white longitudinal meniscal repairs in patients 20 years of age or younger. The American Journal of Sports Medicine. 2011;**39**:1008-1017

[38] Landreau P, Christel P, Djian P. Pathologie ligamentaire du genou. Springer; 2004. XV, 650p

[39] Anderson AF, Anderson CN. Correlation of meniscal and articular cartilage injuries in children and adolescents with timing of anterior cruciate ligament reconstruction. The American Journal of Sports Medicine. 2015;**43**(2):275-281

[40] De Albornoz PM, Forriol F. The meniscal healing process. Muscles, Ligaments and Tendons Journal. 2012;**2**(1):10-18. Print Jan 2012

[41] Chevrier A, Nelea M, Hurtig MB, Hoemann CD, Buschmann MD. Meniscus structure in human, sheep, and rabbit for animal models of meniscus repair. Journal of Orthopaedic Research. 2009;**27**(9):1197-1203

[42] Pujol N, Barbier O, Boisrenoult P, et al. Amount of meniscal resection after failed meniscal repair. The American Journal of Sports Medicine. 2011;**39**:1648-1652

[43] Stein T, Mehling AP, Welsch F, et al. Long-term outcome after arthroscopic meniscal repair versus arthroscopic partial meniscectomy for traumatic meniscal tears. The American Journal of Sports Medicine. 2010;**38**:1542-1548

[44] Paxton ES, Stock MV, Brophy RH. Meniscal repair versus partial meniscectomy: A systematic review comparing reoperation rates and clinical outcomes. Arthroscopy. 2011;**27**:1275-1288

[45] Xu C, Zhao J. A meta-analysis comparing meniscal repair with meniscectomy in the treatment of meniscal tears: The more meniscus, the better outcome? Knee Surgery, Sports Traumatology, Arthroscopy. 2015;**23**(1):164-170

[46] Logan M, Watts M, Owen J, Myers P. Meniscal repair in the elite athlete: Results of 45 repairs with a minimum 5-year follow-up. The American Journal of Sports Medicine. 2009;**37**(6):1131-1134

[47] Buseck MS, Noyes FR. Arthroscopic evaluation of meniscal repairs after anterior cruciate ligament reconstruction and immediate motion. The American Journal of Sports Medicine. 1991;**19**:489-494

[48] Haklar U, Kocaoglu B, Nalbantoglu U, Tuzuner T, Guven O. Arthroscopic repair of radial lateral meniscus tear by double horizontal sutures with inside-outside technique. The Knee. 2008;**15**(5):355-359

[49] Arnoczky SP, Warren RF, McDevitt CA. Meniscal replacement using a cryopreserved allograft. An experimental study in the dog. Clinical Orthopaedics and Related Research. 1990;**252**:121-128

[50] De Girolamo L, Galliera E, Volpi P, Denti M, Dogliotti G, Quaglia A, et al. Why menisci show higher healing rate when repaired during ACL reconstruction? Growth factors release can be the explanation. Knee Surgery, Sports Traumatology, Arthroscopy. 2015;**23**:90-96

[51] Griffin JW, Hadeed MM, Werner BC, Diduch DR, Carson EW,

Miller MD. Platelet-rich plasma in meniscal repair: Does augmentation improve surgical outcomes? Clinical Orthopaedics and Related Research. 2015;**473**(5):1665-1672

[52] Ochi M, Uchio Y, Okuda K, et al. Expression of cytokines after meniscal rasping to promote meniscal healing. Arthroscopy. 2001;**17**:724-731

[53] Shelbourne KD, Gray T. Meniscus tears that can be left in situ, with or without trephination or synovial abrasion to stimulate healing. Sports Medicine and Arthroscopy Review. 2012;**20**:62-67

[54] Haklar U, Donmez F, Basaran SH, Canbora MK. Results of arthroscopic repair of partial- or full-thickness longitudinal medial meniscal tears by single or double vertical sutures using the inside-out technique. The American Journal of Sports Medicine. 2013;**41**(3):596-602

[55] Kozlowski EJ, Barcia AM, Tokish JM. Meniscus repair: The role of accelerated rehabilitation in return to sport. Sports Medicine and Arthroscopy Review. 2012;**20**:121-126

[56] Pabian P, Hanney WJ. Functional rehabilitation after medial meniscus repair in a high school football quarterback: A case report. North American Journal of Sports Physical Therapy. 2008;**3**(3):161-169

[57] Horibe S, Shino K, Nakata K, Maeda A, Nakamura N, Matsumoto N. Second look arthroscopy after meniscal repair. Review of 132 menisci repaired by an arthroscopic inside-out technique. Journal of Bone and Joint Surgery. British Volume (London). 1995;**77**:245-249

[58] Becker R, Brettschneider O, Grobel KH, von Verson R, Starke C. Distraction forces on repaired bucket-handle lesions in the medial meniscus. The American Journal of Sports Medicine. 2006;**34**:1941-1947

[59] Bray RC, Smith JA, Eng MK, Leonard CA, Sutherland CA, Salo PT. Vascular response of the meniscus to injury: Effects of immobilization. Journal of Orthopaedic Research. 2001;**19**:384-390

[60] Lind M, Nielsen T, Faunø P, Lund B, Christiansen SE. Free rehabilitation is safe after isolated meniscus repair: A prospective randomized trial comparing free with restricted rehabilitation regimens. The American Journal of Sports Medicine. 2013;**41**(12):2753-2758

[61] Frizziero A, Ferrari R, Giannotti E, Ferroni C, Poli P, Masiero S. The meniscus tear. State of the art of rehabilitation protocols related to surgical procedures. Muscles, Ligaments and Tendons Journal. 2013;**2**(4):295-301

[62] Kim SG, Nagao M, Kamata K, Maeda K, Nozawa M. Return to sport after arthroscopic meniscectomy on stable knees. BMC Sports Science, Medicine and Rehabilitation. 2013;**5**(1):23. DOI: 10.1186/2052-1847-5-23

[63] Boyd KT, Myers PT. Meniscus preservation; rationale, repair techniques and results. The Knee. 2003;**10**(1):1-11

[64] Turman KA, Diduch DR. Meniscal repair: Indications and techniques. The Journal of Knee Surgery. 2008;**21**(2):154-162

[65] Rodeo SA, Senevirante AM. Arthroscopic meniscal repair using outside-in technique: Indications technique and results. Sports Medicine and Arthroscopy Review. 1999;**7**(1):20-27

[66] Horibe S, Shino K, Nakata K, Maeda A, Nakamura N, Matsumoto N. Second-look arthroscopy after meniscal repair.

Review of 132 menisci repaired by an arthroscopic inside-out technique. Journal of Bone and Joint Surgery. 1995;**77**(2):245-249

[67] Arnoczky SP, Warren RF, Spivak JM. Meniscal repair using an exogenous fibrin clot: An experimental study in dogs. The Journal of Bone and Joint Surgery. American Volume. 1988;**70**:1209-1217

[68] Zhang Z, Arnold JA, Williams T, McCann B. Repairs by trephination and suturing of longitudinal injuries in the avascular area of the meniscus in goats. The American Journal of Sports Medicine. 1995

[69] Zhang Z, Arnold JA. Trephination and suturing of avascular meniscal tears. A clinical study of the trephination procedure. Arthroscopy. 1996;**12**:726-731

[70] Reha Tandoğan N. Menisküs Tamiri: Endikasyon ve Prensipler. Turkish Society of Orthopaedics and Traumatology. 2002;**1**(1)

[71] Kobuna Y, Shirakura K, Niijima M. Meniscal repair using a flap of synovium. An experimental study in the dog. The American Journal of Knee Surgery. 1995;**8**(2):52-55

[72] Kollias SL, Fox JM. Meniscal repair: Where do we from here? Clinics in Sports Medicine. 1996;**15**(3):621-630

[73] Weber RJ, Harris M, Hough AJ. Cell culture of rabbit meniscal fibrochondrocytes: Proliferative and synthetic response to growth factors and ascorbate. Journal of Orthopaedic Research. 1985;**3**:36-42

[74] Spindler KP, Mayes CE, Miller RR. Regional mitogenic response of the meniscus to platelet-derived growth factor (PDGF-AB). Journal of Orthopaedic Research. 1995;**13**:201-207

[75] Barber FA. Meniscus repair aftercare. Sports Medicine and Arthroscopy Review. 1999;**7**(1):43-47

[76] Verdonk R, Verdonk P, Huysse W, Forsyth R, Heinrichs EL. Tissue ingrowth after implantation of a novel, biodegradable polyurethane scaffold for treatment of partial meniscal lesions. The American Journal of Sports Medicine. 2011;**39**(4):774-782

[77] Zaffagnini S, Grassi A, Marcheggiani Muccioli GM, Holsten D, Bulgheroni P, et al. Two-year clinical results of lateral collagen meniscus implant: A multicenter study. Arthroscopy. 2015;**31**(7):1269-1278

[78] Gentile NE, Stearns KM, Brown EH, Rubin JP, Boninger ML, Dearth CL, et al. Targeted rehabilitation after extracellular matrix scaffold transplantation for the treatment of volumetric muscle loss. American Journal of Physical Medicine & Rehabilitation. 2014;**93**(11 Suppl 3): S79-S87

[79] Gür S, Janousek AT, Fu FH. Allogreft menisküs transplantasyonu. Acta Orthopaedica et Traumatologica Turcica. 1997;**31**:429-436

[80] Kim JM, Jeon BS, Lee CR, Lim SJ, Kim KA, Bin SI. Comparison of postoperative magnetic resonance imaging and second look arthroscopy for evaluating meniscal allograft transplantation. Arthroscopy. 2015;**31**(5):859-866

[81] Sonnery-Cottet B, Archbold P, Thaunat M, Carnesecchi O, Tostes M, Chambat P. Rapid chondrolysis of the knee after partial lateral meniscectomy in professional athletes. The Knee. 2014;**21**(2):504-508

[82] Lee DH, Kim SB, Kim TH, Cha EJ, Bin SI. Midterm outcomes after meniscal allograft transplantation:

Comparison of cases with extrusion versus without extrusion. The American Journal of Sports Medicine. 2010;**38**:247-254

[83] Matava MJ. Meniscal allograft transplantation: A systematic review. Clinical Orthopaedics and Related Research. 2007;**455**:142-157

Section 2

Arthroscopic Evaluation of the Meniscus

Chapter 2

Arthroscopic Anatomy of the Knee Joint and Portals

Vaso Kecojevic, Vladimir Harhaji and Srđan Ninković

Abstract

Knee arthroscopy is one of the most used operative treatments in orthopedic surgery. The first knee arthroscopy was performed by Prof. K. Takagi, from Tokyo, Japan, in 1920. With further improvement, he made the first black and white photos of the inside of the knee (1932) and, soon, the first color photos (1939). Independently from Takagi, Dr. Eugen Bircher from Arau, Switzerland, in 1921 published the results of 20 "arthro-endoscopies," and that was the first time the word "arthroscopy" was mentioned in literature. In New York, USA, Dr. Michael Burman described in detail the incision points and technique of joint spreading that we use today. In 1957, Dr. Masaki Watanabe published the first Atlas of Arthroscopy. The first Arthroscopy Course in English language was held in Philadelphia, USA, in 1972. The International Arthroscopy Association, with Dr. Watanabe as president, was established in 1974. In clinical knee arthroscopy, the following division proved to be very useful: the medial compartment, the lateral compartment, the central part or central pivot, and the femoropatelar compartment. In this chapter, the normal anatomy of each of this part will be described in detail, with the descriptions of basic knee arthroscopy portals.

Keywords: knee, arthroscopy, anatomy, portals

1. Introduction

The anatomical definition of the knee is determined by the fact that the knee connects the upper and lower leg, made up of the knee joint, the patelofemoral joint, and the proximal tibiofibular joint, and the soft tissues surrounding them. In the frontal plane of the femur and tibia, an angle of 174° is made, which makes the physiological valgus of the knee. In women, valgus and recurvatum are slightly higher. The borders of the joint are on the buttock, the line that passes at 2–3 cm above the base of the patella, and on the lower leg, the circular line that passes directly below the tibial tubercle [1].

Anatomically speaking, the knee consists of bone and soft tissue structures, which built four topographic regions. In clinical knee arthroscopy, the following division proved to be very useful: the medial part consists of a medial femoral condyle, medial tibial plateau, medial meniscus, and medial part of the capsule and ligaments. The lateral part consists of a lateral femoral condyle, lateral tibial plateau, lateral meniscus, and lateral ligaments and capsules, including arch complex (lig. arcuatum). The central part or central pivot is composed of an intercondylar notch, which comprises crossed ligaments, anterior and posterior intercondylar

IntechOpen

field of the tibia (lower part of the attachment of crossed ligaments of the knee), and intercondylar eminences and tubercles. The femoropatelar part consists of a femoropatelar joint, an infrapatellar fat tissue, a patellar ligament, and a quadriceps tendon and normally presents medial and lateral patellar plicas and suprapatellar recess [2, 3].

2. Surgical anatomy of the knee

2.1 Medial compartment

2.1.1 Anterior third

Outside, superficially through the articular capsule, the horizontal part of the m. vastus medialis (m. vastus medialis obliquus) is provided. The attachment of the pes anserinus (m. sartorisu, m. gracilis, m. semitendinosus) extends from the back and down in the upper two-thirds of the tibia. The medial patellar retinaculum extends from the upper two-thirds of the medial part of the patella and is attached to the outside of the medial femoral condyle. Medial longitudinal patellar retinaculum originates from a wide base between the patella, the medial vastus, and the upper attachment of the medial collateral ligament and descends to the upper part of the tibia where it is attached behind the pes anserinus and in front and above the attachment of the medial collateral ligament. Both retinacula cover the anterior part of the joint, and their fibers come from the medial vastus and quadriceps tendon, which allows them to function as dynamic stabilizers. The individual fibers of the medial longitudinal retinaculum are drowned in the medial collateral ligament, and the other is joined to the tendon of the pes anserinus and extends to the popliteal fascia. Deep fibers extend beyond the superficial fascia to the medial collateral ligament and semimembranosus. Retinacula controls the movements of the patella toward the femur (limits the lateral deviation) and equalizes the pressure of the lateral and medial joint surface of the patella and the internal rotation of the tibia (via m. vastus medialis obliquus and patellar ligament). The pes anserinus-conjoined tendon, by its superficial position, acts as a ligament-muscle protector of the medial side of the joint in flexion and extension. Functionally, it represents an active duplicative of the medial collateral ligament [2, 3].

2.1.2 Middle third

In the middle third, the dominant structure is the medial collateral ligament as a deep tensioner under the tendon of the pes anserinus. It extends sloping down and backward from the lateral femoral condyle to the upper tibia. It consists of two thin layers, structurally different. The deep layer consists mainly of femoro-meniscal and menisco-tibial fibers. The superficial layer is structurally separate from the medial meniscus and has nothing to do with it, except in the back part where the superficial and deep layer joins and builds a posterior oblique ligament, which is attached to the posterior horn of the medial meniscus. The fibers are further arranged to “divide” the ligament into the triangles so that they are tilted selectively toward the position of the knee. This reduces the change in force, e.g., the longest fibers are tight in flexion and the shortest in the extension. In moderate flexion of the knee, all the fibers are loose and allow rotatory knee movements.

The upper third of the ligament is attached to the femur, and the lower for the tibia. During the flexion that begins with the rolling of the femoral condyle, the front fibers move backward through the femoral and tibial surfaces. That's why the ligament must be freely movable in these places (as well as through the medial meniscus) to glide over the bones and must not have a deep-coated attachment.

The superficial fibers are connected in the posterior part with the deep fibers (and built posterior oblique ligament) and with fibers of m. semimembranosus, and therefore the superficial fibers of the ligaments are dynamized by this muscle, especially in the position of flexion. The attachment of the remainder of the fiber to the fascia and tendon of the adductor magnus contributes to the further dynamization of the ligament. The relationship of the m. vastus medialis to the medial patellar retinaculum has already been described. A passive, firm bone attachment is present in the deeper parts of the ligament. Superficial fibers are largely dynamically bound to muscles, so passive instability can be compensated by a good muscular function, and the fibers can adequately adapt to great demands and work [2–4].

2.1.3 Posterior third

The posterior medial third of the knee—the "semimembranosus angle"—represents a functionally important part. It is separated from the medial collateral ligament in spite of the topographical close relationship. The structurally and functionally key element of this angle is the lig. posterior obliquus, which extends between the tendons of adductor magnus and semimembranosus. The main active rear stabilizer is semimembranosus muscle, which stabilizes the knee posteriorly. Semimembranosus muscle is attached to the posteromedial angle by five separate finger extensions. The first two, which go directly to the lig. obliquus posterior and climb straight through the posterior capsule as lig. popliteus obliquus, make semimembranosus an active stabilizer of the posteromedial angle. The attachments are arranged so that at least one is taut in every position of the flexion and directs the traction in the appropriate direction to give the angle of flexion. The finer are the backward fibers that flow from the m. vastus medialis. At maximal extension, the angle of semimembranosus is below the maximum tension due to the associated posteromedial sliding of the medial femoral condyle. In extension, semimembranosus helps in stabilization of the entire medial side. In 90° flexion, it has an additional role in the transmission of tension to the free capsule-ligament fibers and stabilizes the knee to prevent external rotation [2, 4].

2.1.4 Medial meniscus

The structural element of the medial compartment, from the anterior to the posterior third, is medial meniscus. It has a crescent shape, it is narrower in the front, and it extends to the rear. The free edge is facing the knee joint, and the rim is attached to the articular capsule. In the anterior third, it is relatively narrow, it is attached to the tibial plateau with a fibrous bundle that extends the meniscus anteriorly, and there is also a medial part that secures the anterolateral part of the meniscus to the anterior intercondylar area. The anterior horns of the medial and lateral meniscus are connected by the fibrous bridge that makes the transversal knee ligament. The medial patello-meniscal ligament extends from the anterior edge of the medial meniscus to the patella. In the middle third, the meniscus is still narrow. At the outer edge, there are femoral-meniscal and tibial-meniscal fibers (coronary ligament) but without an attachment to the medial collateral ligament. In the posterior third, the meniscus is spreading to the posterior horn. The femoromeniscal fibers and the coronary ligament join to the posterior oblique ligament and fix the last horn of the meniscus for the ligament. The fibers at the lower part of the posterior horn link the meniscus for the posterior intercondylar area. The horn must be firmly attached to the coronary and anteromedial collateral ligament in order to participate in anteroposterior stabilization and perform the essential role of a stress-transfer gearbox ("brakes" that limit the frontal movement of the tibia and the last displacement of the femur). This function is only possible if the femoro-meniscal part of the posterior oblique ligament and the posterior horn of the medial meniscus are intact (femoral condyle can "settle down"), and the semimembranosus attachment is not damaged (to maintain rotatory stability). ACL works synergistically with the posterior oblique ligament, by both of them tightening during the front translation of the tibia. Approximately 80% of ACL ruptures are associated with lesions of medial ligaments (the posterior oblique ligament, medial collateral ligament) [5–9].

2.2 Lateral compartment

The outer compartment has relatively weak passive stabilizers. Active stabilizers are dominant and those are: iliotibial tract (m. tensor fasciae latae and m. gluteus maximus), m. biceps femoris, and m. popliteus. The relative dominance of dynamic structures is in correlation with a higher degree of displacement during flexion (m. biceps femoris, m. popliteus, and m. tensor fasciae latae). In the lateral part, three subregions are described.

2.2.1 Anterior third

Similar to the medial part, characteristic are lateral superficial and longitudinal patellar retinacula. The attachment of the lateral longitudinal retinaculum is somewhat different from the medial, due to the more limited extension of m. vastus lateralis, as well as due to the presence of an iliotibial band outside the retinaculum. A part of the fibers of the iliotibial band ends at the lateral femoral condyle, the part extends to the patella, and the main part goes to Gerdy's tubercle. Lateral patellar retinaculum is attached to the iliotibial band with multiple fibers, and from there it extends to the patella. The lateral longitudinal retinaculum fibers originate from three different sites, patella, m. vastus lateralis, and iliotibial band, and some extend (to the lateral femoral epicondyle or tibia—Gerdy's tubercle) from the lateral iliotibial band. The lateral longitudinal patellar retinaculum is attached to the medial portion of Gerdy's tubercle and adjacent proximal to tibia parts.

Both lateral retinacula are dynamically linked to m. vastus lateralis, tensor fasciae latae (iliotibial tract), and gluteus maximus muscle (iliotibial tract). The main role of lateral retinaculum is to maintain the femoro-patellar sliding (by preventing the medial deviation of the patella) and the equalization of the pressure between the lateral and the medial half of the patella.

Due to its position and attachment, the iliotibial tract acts as a "lateral femoro-tibial collateral ligament" and plays an important role in the function of the femoro-tibial joint. Its dynamic parts end up on the lateral femoral condyle (Kaplan's complex fibers at the Krakow spot) and proximal tibia (Gerdy's tubercle). The passive fibers are placed forward and deeper and establish a firm connection between the lateral condyle and Gerdy's tubercle, so they are often distinguished as an "anterolateral femoro-tibial ligament."

The iliotibial band synergistically works with two groups of muscles. In the position from 0 to 40° of flexion, it moves forward with respect to the axis of rotation and thus supports the extensor muscles. By increasing the flexion, it slides backward through the lateral epicondyle (behind the axis of flexion) and becomes synergistic to the flexor muscle group when the flexion exceeds 40° (the launch of the iliotibial band via the femoral epicondyle plays an important role in the existence of the pivot shift). The iliotibial band functionally helps in anterolateral rotatory stability by fixing the knee toward the lateral opening (stress varus). It also stabilizes the lateral tibial plateau, preventing sliding forward with rotary movements.

In the deep layer of the front and middle third, there is a joint capsule. It consists of a synovial coat, and, in the absence of reinforcement by the ligament fibers, it is very stretchable. Only the lateral patello-meniscal ligament fibers pass from the outer edge of the meniscus to the patella and are sometimes incorporated into the capsule. The ligament serves as a receptor for the reflex stabilization of femoro-patellar and femoro-tibial movements, analogously to the medial menisco-patellar ligament. The anterior part of the deep articular capsule is freely movable in relation to the iliotibial band. It is covered with fatty tissue that is absorbed into the infrapatellar fat tissue. It is firmly attached to the edge of the lateral meniscus. The fibers of the transferal ligament of the knee pass from the anterior horn of the lateral meniscus to the opposite side [2, 3].

2.2.2 Middle third

Structurally and functionally, the middle and posterior thirds are closely related. Most elements show hierarchical arrangement from the front to the rear or vice versa.

The most superficial in this area is the wide tendon of biceps femoris muscle. It extends downward and forward in the outer part of the last third and connects on the head of the fibula with two arms: the back, the greater part, and the front (middle attachment of the biceps tendon together with the fibular collateral ligament). Trauma is a common cause of bone tendon avulsion, and also high muscular strain can cause dislocation of the fibular head. The biceps femoris tendon is attached to the tibia by the extensions that pass over and below the lateral collateral ligament. Biceps femoris muscle is an important stabilizer of varus angulation in extended knee and internal rotation in flexion (more specifically, the short head of biceps femoris muscle is the main antagonist of the popliteal muscle and thus the internal rotation). In addition to being an important external rotator, biceps femoris muscle is also a flexor, due to the position behind the axis of flexion.

The lateral collateral ligament descends back and forth from the femoral condyle to the fibula's head. It is smaller than the medial collateral ligament but can be identified as a separate structure. It contributes to passive stabilization of the outside of the knee, and synergist is to the posterior cruciate ligament (PCL). Deep and completely separated from the lateral collateral ligament is the popliteal muscle tendon, which starts from the lateral femoral condyle and descends backward where it connects with the body of the popliteal muscle in the last third of the lateral section. The articular capsule is very thin and is not firmly attached to other structural collagen elements. It is noticeable that there is no anatomical connection with the lateral meniscus, whose edge is freely moving in the middle third of the outer compartment [2, 3].

2.2.3 Posterior third

In the posterior part of the lateral side dominates, structurally and functionally, the popliteal muscle. More superficial are the fibers of the oblique popliteal ligament. The fibers end up on the fabella or, if this does not exist, extend outer and upward to the attachment of the lateral head of the gastrocnemius muscle. In this way, the fabella and the oblique popliteal ligament are bound structurally and functionally to the lateral tendon of gastrocnemius muscle. In this area, the deep part of the muscle tendon strengthens the joint capsule. Distally, the fabella joint capsule and the tendon of gastrocnemius muscle are separated. On the distal part of the fabella, the arch ligament (which is a tendon extension from popliteal muscle) and a fabello-fibular ligament are attached (Vallois). These extensions emphasize the role of the fabella as the point where stress is transmitted (although it is present in only about 20% of the population).

The arch ligament extends from the posterior part of the tibia and the head of the fibula to the middle of the joint capsule. Some fibers are projecting to the fabella, but it also receives fibers from m. popliteus (the beginning of the tendon is branching) and allows the muscle to tighten the ligament to the fabella. The deep part of the ligament is attached to the posterior horn of the lateral meniscus with the tendons of the popliteal muscle, so popliteal muscle actively pulls the meniscus during flexion until the femoral condyle is rotated backward.

The popliteal muscle is originated from the posteromedial tibial surface and is initially parallel to the arch ligament. After giving extensions for the arch ligament and the posterior horn of the lateral meniscus, the muscle continues laterally forward and upward. In a deep layer, the tendon passes behind the arch ligament; enters the popliteal aperture; then goes over the outer part of the upper tibia, below the lateral collateral ligament; and is attached to the lateral femoral condyle. The tendon has the thickness of the pencil. Besides attachments to the arch ligament, the lateral meniscus, and the femur, there are also deep direct tendon attachments for the posterior joint capsule. Popliteal muscle also acts as an internal rotator of the tibia in flexion.

The posterior part of the capsule is reinforced with fibers which are sometimes referred to as the posterolateral collateral ligament. The fibers enter the capsule as a ligament, and they are almost parallel with the popliteal tendon and are attached to the posterior horn of the lateral meniscus and to the tibia. The most important active stabilizer of the posterolateral angle is the popliteal muscle with its deep attachments.

The posterior part of the lateral meniscus is directly linked to the posterior capsule, the popliteal tendon, and the arch popliteal ligament (most common site of avulsions and ruptures). Popliteal muscle actively pulls and puts the lateral meniscus under the lateral femoral condyle during flexion and prevents the meniscus from incarceration under the condyle. The popliteal aperture gives more space that is necessary for the lateral meniscus for its high mobility (thus reducing the incidence of rupture in this area). In the popliteal aperture, the tendon is completely separated from the meniscus. The posterior horn of the meniscus is tied to the central part of the joint. The posterior menisco-femoral ligament (Wrisberg) attaches the meniscus to the posterior intercondylar area of the tibia, while the anterior menisco-femoral ligament (Humphry) attaches the front part of the posterior horn to the posterior part of an anterior intercondylar area.

There is a symmetrical, functionally connected triad of elements of the posteromedial and posterolateral parts of the joint. On the medial side, there are the posterior horn of the medial meniscus, the posterior oblique ligament, and the semimembranosus muscle and on the lateral side posterior horn of the lateral meniscus, arch complex, and popliteal muscle. Further symmetry is observed in relation to the synergistic function. The internal posteromedial elements are in functional correlation with ACL (combined lesion in 80% of cases) and posterolateral angle with PCL (again, combined lesions in 80% of cases) [2, 3].

2.3 Central part (central pivot)

The dominant structures of the central pivot are cruciate ligaments, anterior (ACL) and posterior (PCL). Both ligaments together form a line of femoral condyles and kinematic laws of joint movements. The anterior third of the central pivot, bounded by the intercondylar area of the tibia and the intercondylar groove of the femur, is the site of the attachment of the anterior horns of medial and lateral meniscus and the transverse ligament of the knee. Between them, the relatively wide space of the intercondylar area is occupied by a tibial attachment of the ACL. With the extended knee, the ACL extends vertically over the intercondylar groove to the attachment back on the lateral femoral condyle. In hyperextension it retracts under the vault of the groove in the intercondylar notch called "Grant's groove." At this point the ligament can be twisted or even ruptured if it is too tight on the groove. Grant's groove is a measure of the width of the ACL. In the knee flexion, the ACL comes in a horizontal position and is closely related to the PCL at the point where they cross, directly above the vascular pedicle.

ACL stabilizes the tibia toward the frontal translation relative to the femur. The elements of the posteromedial angle of semimembranosus and anterolateral femoro-tibial ligament also act synergistically. Approximately one-third of the capacity of the anterior stabilization is due to ACL, and the remaining are of two structural elements (the isolated rupture of the ACL leaves two-thirds of the capacity intact). The structure of the ligament is such that it almost never transmits load through the entire surface; individual fibers are loaded selectively during a particular movement or in a particular position of the joint. Anteromedial fibers are most affected when the knee is almost extended, posterolateral fibers when the knee is flexed in a higher degree, and intermediate fibers stabilize the internal rotation, during which the fibers of the ligaments rotate.

ACL vascularization comes from the branches of the middle geniculate artery. This blood vessel connects the ACL and PCL at the crossing point. The artery enters the ACL from the subcortical web, but does not feed the whole ligament but only the sites of attachment.

Both cruciate ligaments have a common frontal synovial sheath. In spite of the intra-articular position, both ligaments are extrasynovial. The common synovia originates from the crossed "central pivot," and it is vascularized by the branches of the middle geniculate artery.

PCL is better vascularized; it receives four branches of the middle geniculate artery that are arranged throughout the entire length of the ligament. Its origin from a wide area on the medial part of the medial femoral condyle passes downward and backward and is attached to the posterior intercondylar area of the tibia on a small surface. During knee extension it is relatively flat and rises during knee flexion, but it does not have the risk of collapsing under the front edge of the intercondylar groove. After achieving vertical position during flexion, the PCL becomes the central point of the knee rotation and has a significant stabilization effect. The only synergistic effect in the flexion has a quadriceps femoris muscle. In the knee extension, because of PCL-like orientation, the posterior oblique ligament and posteromedial capsule are acting synergistically, and they rupture together in the trauma. Like the ACL, the PCL consists of three strands of fibers that are loaded depending on the position of the joint. Posteromedial fibers tighten in the extension and limit hyperextension (their attachment is furthest on the intercondylar area). The central and anterolateral bundles are tense at medium and full flexion (their attachment is on the outside of the posterior intercondylar area, near the lateral meniscus). In addition to other functions, the PCL is the posterior translation stopper, although in the case of internal rotation, this role can be partly taken by the Humphry and Wrisberg menisco-femoral ligaments that are tightened in that position (and therefore may mask the posterior instability in the position of the internal rotation of the knee). On the medial side, PCL is connected by fibers with the posterior horn of the medial meniscus.

Intercondylar eminence of the tibia is the basic axis of rotation of the knees in small and middle flexion. It is covered with a thick, strong layer of cartilage and is located between the medial surfaces of the femoral condyles, which are also covered with cartilage. The posterior part of the meniscal cartilage, which differs in hardness, thickness, and resistance, can act as a duplication of intercondylar eminence. The axial role of eminence in moderate flexion is important for guiding an articular surface in varus, valgus, or rotatory loads and for the absorption of compressive forces, especially since the peripheral joint structures in this position is loosened.

Cruciate ligaments can protect the joint from varus and valgus stress by assuming the role of "inner" collateral ligaments for a particular femoral condyle in case the collateral ligaments are ruptured. The next important role of cruciate ligaments is in the mechanism of terminal locking of the knee. This automatic terminal rotation is caused by the position of the cruciate ligaments and the unequal length of the femoral condyles. The lateral femoral condyle, due to its smaller length, is first placed on the tibial plateau and ends its rolling, while the longer medial condyle continues rolling [2, 3, 8, 10, 11].

2.4 Patello-femoral compartment

The central structure of the patellofemoral joint is patella, a sesamoid bone which, although mobile, is a fixed point for the attachment of ligaments and tendons. Analogue to the fabella in the posterolateral corner of the flexor side, the patella is a key point for forces transmitted from multiple directions: longitudinal traction forces across the quadriceps tendon and patellar ligament and transverse traction forces through the menisco-patellar ligaments and transverse retinacula. Accordingly, the function of the patella depends entirely on the action of quadriceps femoris muscle. The upper part of the patella (base) has grown in the quadriceps tendon, extra-articular, and has no joint surface. Intra-articular space extends from the tip of the patella to the quadriceps tendon, along the front side of the femur, forming a suprapatellar recess. The lower, articular surface of the patella does not fit smoothly on the trochlea all over its surface in flexion or extension. The medial part of the patella is covered with a thin layer of cartilage, and the joint surface is incorrectly curved and does not fully attach to the medial part of the trochlea; this occasionally creates a free space between the hinged surfaces in which the synovia retract, which contributes to a more uniform distribution of loads. The outer part of the patella corresponds to the outer part of the trochlea. In the extension of the knee, the patella is completely attached to the femoral joint surface. In full flexion, the lower part of the patella lies in front of the condylar part of the femorotibial joint. Sulcus terminalis separates the femoral patellar surface, with relatively high edges, especially laterally, from the area of the femorotibial joint. The distal part of the patella, as well as the upper end, grew into the ligament tissue—the patellar ligament. Posteriorly, there is a well-vascular infrapatellar fat tissue (Hoffa). It is held in place by the patellar ligaments, bilateral longitudinal retinaculum, and infrapatellar synovial plaque (odd structure centrally positioned and posteriorly up to the roof of the intercondylar groove). Movement of the patella is consistent with a fine control mechanism in which medial and lateral patello-meniscal ligaments play an important role (receptor function). This explains the identical clinical picture of medial patellar chondropathy and the lesion of the medial meniscus.

The function of the patello-femoral joint is completely dependent on the function of quadriceps. The action of the muscle causes sliding of the patella through the trochlea. This action exerts a greater pressure on the lateral part of the condyle than on the medial, since the main vector of the quadriceps force is lateral (Q angle). This causes a slight posterior movement of the lateral femoral condyle associated with the internal rotation of the tibia. Vastus medialis muscle and vastus medialis obliquus muscles are antagonists of these forces and take the patella medially.
The large contact pressure of the patella on the lateral femoral condyle occurs in

conjunction with angulation and external rotation, and vastus obliquus muscle is again an antagonist. Conversely, the patellar pressure on the medial femoral condyle increases during angulation in the internal rotation, and vastus lateralis muscle performs an antagonistic traction role. In the neutral rotation position, the lateral and medial vastus muscle acts equally as an agonist and antagonist, resulting in constant pressure changes on different contact surfaces in the medial, lateral, proximal, and distal directions. The normal mobility of the patella is based on a separate action of the different parts of quadriceps. A small disorder in this complex functional sequence leads rapidly to the decompensation of a finely balanced system. This particularly applies to the medial joint surface, where even moderate disorder rapidly leads to abnormalities in nutrition and diffusion [2, 3].

2.5 Menisci

Menisci represented a pair of the C-shaped and wedge cartilages interposed between the femur and tibia in the knee joint.

Menisci play an important role in the distribution of loads, shock absorption, joint stability, and lubrication of joint surfaces. Histologically, they are built from three different types of tissue. At the cross section, the outer part consists of a thick connective tissue that contains nerve endings and is abundantly bled. The middle part is predominantly fibrocartilaginous with fibers of different tensions. The central tissue is predominantly hyaline and contains fewer fibers and blood vessels than the more superficial fibrous tissue. The inner part of the meniscus consists of a pure hyaline cartilage that is avascular and without innervation.

Special importance is attributed to the meniscus architecture. The external parts are partially integrated into the capsuloligamentar system. Some fiber bundles are arranged in arches whose base is directed toward the inside of the joint. In the outer third, the fibers are parallel and in the inner part are more radial. The chemical structure also varies, in the fibrous connective tissue of the outer third, pre-type collagen type I and type III; there are also types V and VI. Elastin and proteoglycans are less represented but functionally relevant. Hyaline cartilage in the inner part consists of collagen type II and proteoglycan. Shorter-chain collagens (type V, IX, XI), as well as different matrix proteins (tenascin and chain proteins), are less represented.

The middle third is histologically and chemically distinct, with a defined topographic difference that causes changes from superficial to deep parts of the meniscus [7, 9, 12, 13].

2.6 Joint capsule and synovia

The structure of the articular capsule shows significant local variations. In some places it has grown into a periarticular ligament system and forms a very strong, mechanically stable layer. In other places, the capsule makes only a thin synovial membrane with surrounding fat and fibrous tissue.

Synovia (synovial membrane, also known as stratum synoviale) consists of two morphologically different tissues. The first (intima) is a superficial cell layer that includes an articulate cavity. By its characteristics, it is epithelial, with a thickness of three to four cells. Between the cells are frequent jaws that open in a subintimal layer of loose connective tissue, which contains abundance of lymph and blood capillaries and numerous scattered fat cells.

Cells of synovial intima do not form a continuous basal membrane that separates the epithelial from the subepithelial connective tissue. Morphologically, three types of cells are distinguished: type A (or type M for “macrophages similar”) whose cytoplasm contains a developed Golgi apparatus, a lot of vacuoles, and lysosomal bubbles but a scarcely rough endoplasmic reticulum and long cell prolongation.

Type B (or F of "fibroblasts similar") contains abundant coarse endoplasmic reticulum but a little vacuum, lysosomal bubbles, and Golgi's lamellas. Cellular attachments are poorly developed. Mixed cell type (sometimes called AB) is also described. Synoviale cells are responsible for the formation of hyaluronic acid, glycosaminoglycan, and some glycoproteins of synovial fluid. Thanks to numerous vesicles, they have the ability of phagocytosis of particles from synovial fluid—this is attributed mainly to M cells. A significant portion of the synovial fluid protein passes from the subintimendous connective tissue directly through the intercellular channels into the synovial fluid. Most proteins are micromolecular plasma proteins that can diffuse through the walls of the capillary from the blood plasma into the intercellular space of the subintimal connective tissue. Free nerve endings were not found in the subintimal region, although there are fibers of the autonomic nervous system that undergo the advent of blood vessels. In deeper layers away from the intima, the number of collagen fibers (stratum fibrosum) increases, in which articular capsules give the characteristics of the ligaments and supply the capsule with numerous nerve fibers, for the transmission of pain, along with blood vessels. This layer establishes numerous structural contacts with periarticular ligaments and creates strong enhancements in some parts of the capsule [7].

3. Basic portals for knee arthroscopy

A patient scheduled for knee arthroscopy is placed on the operative table with the leg planned for arthroscopy placed on the leg holder and opposite leg on side holder (**Figures 1** and **2**). Arthroscopy could be done in general, regional, or local anesthesia, with or without tourniquet. Landmarks for arthroscopy are the patella, patellar ligament, and upper edge of the tibial plateau. The basic portals are anterolateral and anteromedial, and auxiliary portals are suprapatellar medial and lateral, central, posteromedial, and posterolateral (**Figure 3**). Knee arthroscopy starts by making anterolateral portal [2, 3]. The entry point is localized by palpation. The thumb is placed to the soft tissue groove in triangle that is formed by lateral border of patellar ligament, upper lateral part of the tibial plateau, and tip of the patella. Knee is flexed. Above the thumb and near the patellar ligament, we place a 1.2 gauge needle (**Figure 4**). With the tip of the needle, we try to reach a lateral tibial plateau. After pulling the needle out, the skin incision is made at the point that is marked by the needle. Making 0.5–1 cm horizontal incision is a good way to avoid cutting the meniscus. Incision is pointed in 45° angle to the frontal plane. After the incision is made, Kellys clamp is introduced through it in the same direction (**Figure 5**). After touching the medial condyle, the clamp is turned parallel to the condyles and pushed medially, while it can be palpated under the skin on medial side (**Figure 6**). While pulling the clamp back, soft tissue is spreading with Kelly's clamp in a manner to open and close it. The next step is introducing the 4 mm scope in the same manner. Then, slightly extend the knee and hold it in valgus (**Figure 7**). When the medial meniscus is in the field of view, the anteromedial portal is prepared. The entry point should be close to the patellar tendon on the medial border (**Figure 8**). The needle is introduced again from the medial side. We could make a pressure to the skin by the finger looking inside the joint by scope to determine the appropriate entry point. After the needle is visualized in the joint, the skin incision is made. By the visual control, the knife is then used to make the skin incision and to avoid damage of the cartilage or meniscus. Through the anteromedial portal, the probe is introduced in the joint (**Figure 9**).

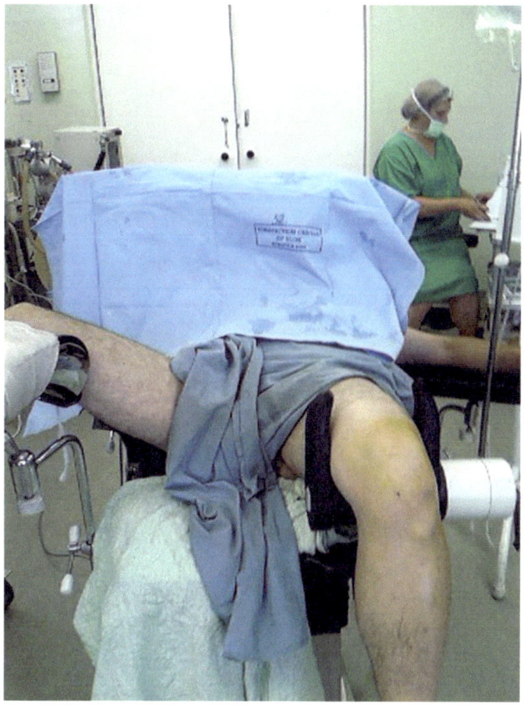

Figure 1.
Knee arthroscopy preparation: Placing the patient on the operative table – frontal view.

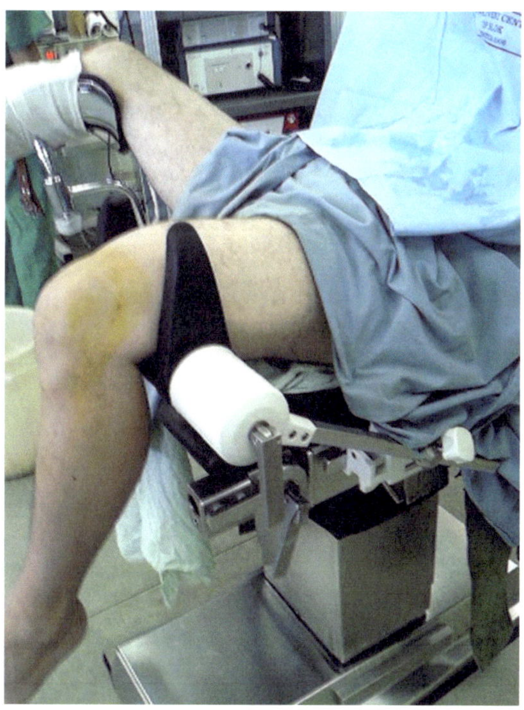

Figure 2.
Knee arthroscopy preparation: Placing the patient on the operative table – side view.

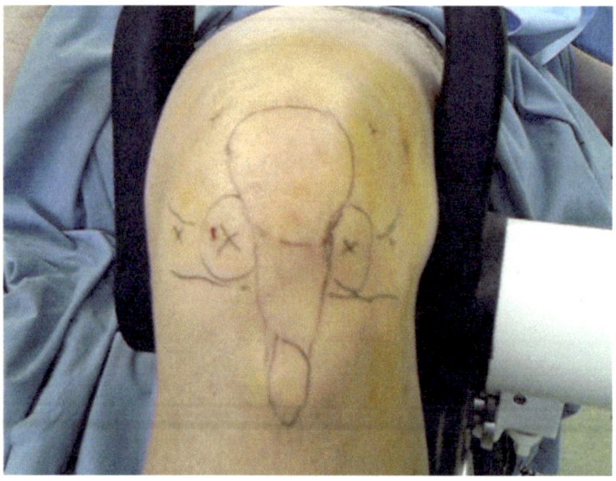

Figure 3.
Basic portals and auxiliary portals are marked on the knee.

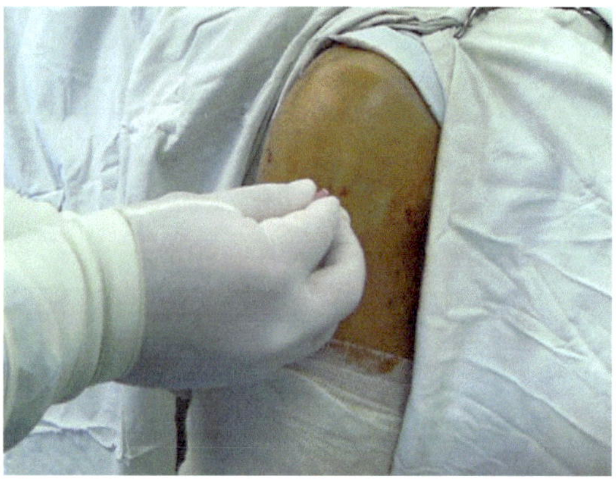

Figure 4.
1.2 gauge needle is placed near the patellar ligament.

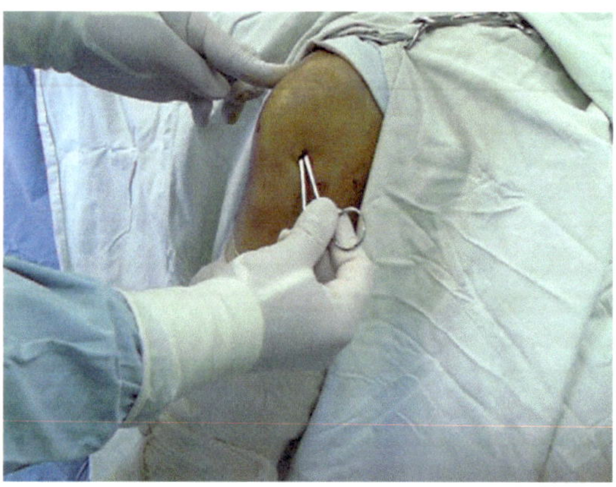

Figure 5.
Kelly's clamp introduced through the horizontal incision (45° angle to the frontal plane).

Examination begins with the suprapatellar recess, then medial compartment, intercondylar notch, and lateral compartment. For placing scope in the suprapatellar recess, the knee has to be extended, and the patella is free to be moved. The main structure in the recess is the so-called suprapatellar plication, which is a white

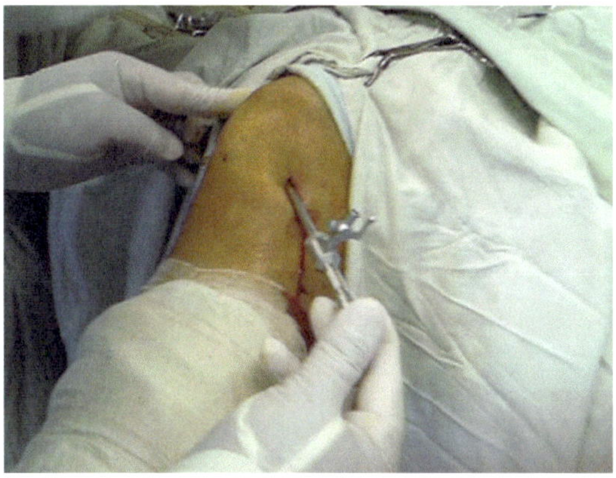

Figure 6.
The clamp is turned parallel to the condyles and pushed medially.

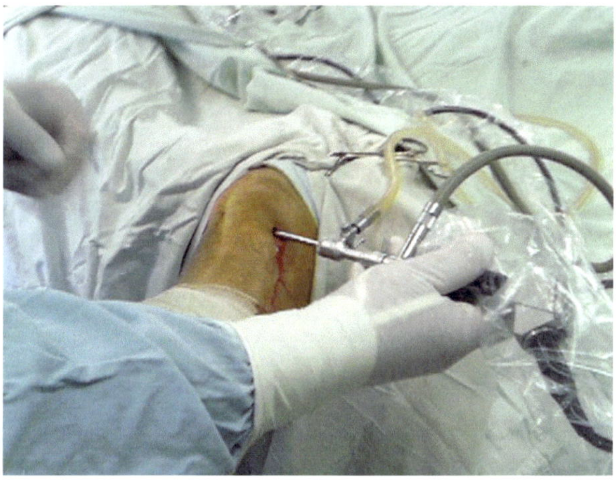

Figure 7.
While pulling the clamp back, soft tissue is spread with Kelly's clamp; then, the 4 mm scope is introduced in the same manner.

band of connective tissue, sometimes separating the recess in two compartments, and can cause the symptoms like pain and snapping. The synovium is orange and red colored and we can see small blood vessels (**Figure 10**). Recess is often placed where we could find loose bodies (**Figure 11**). After examining recess, slightly pull the camera to see the femoral trochlea. The cartilage is white, shiny, and smooth. By rotating the optical for 90°, we can see articular surface of the patella, with the same characteristics (**Figure 12**). Then, slide with the scope medially. At that point we can see cartilage border of the medial femoral condyle and the soft tissue that covers the medial epicondyle. By flexing the knee, the medial collateral ligament can be identified. Sliding down in the field of vision appears the menisco-capsular junction, well vascularized, and we can clearly identify the medial meniscus as white semilunar structure with the inner edge free. Above is the visualized part of the medial femoral condyle, and beneath is the medial tibial plateau. Healthy meniscus is white, smooth, with sharp inner edge, and in full length connected to the capsule (**Figure 13**). Placing the scope beneath the femoral condyle, we should see the attachment of the posterior horn of the medial meniscus (**Figure 14**). The knee should be positioned in semiflexion and valgus. By extending and flexing the

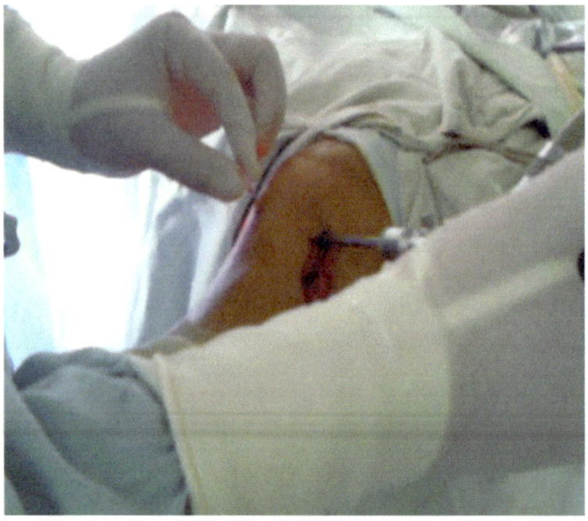

Figure 8.
Anteromedial portal is prepared. The entry point should be close to the patellar tendon on the medial border.

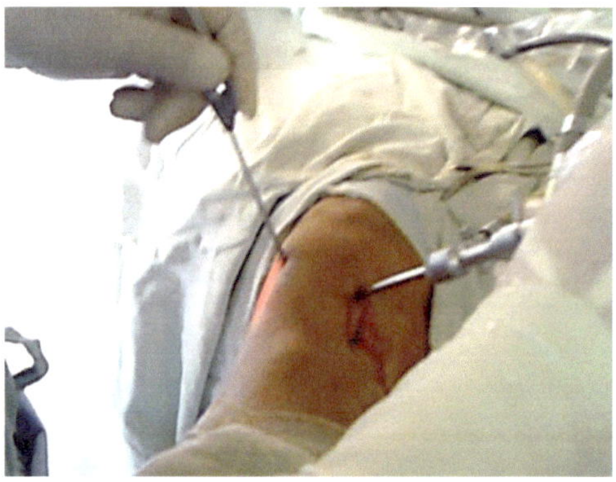

Figure 9.
Through the anteromedial portal, the probe is introduced in the joint.

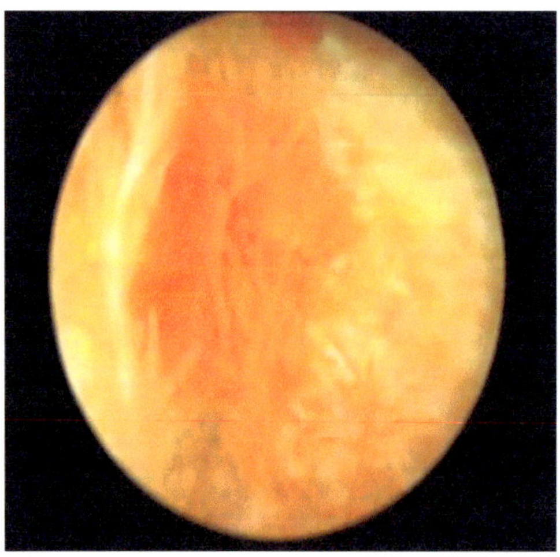

Figure 10.
The synovium is orange and red colored and we can see small blood vessels.

knee, we could examine the whole cartilage of the medial femoral condyle, and next is the intercondylar notch. The main structure is the ACL; it is represented like a white, pale band that arises from the anterior intercondylar area and goes

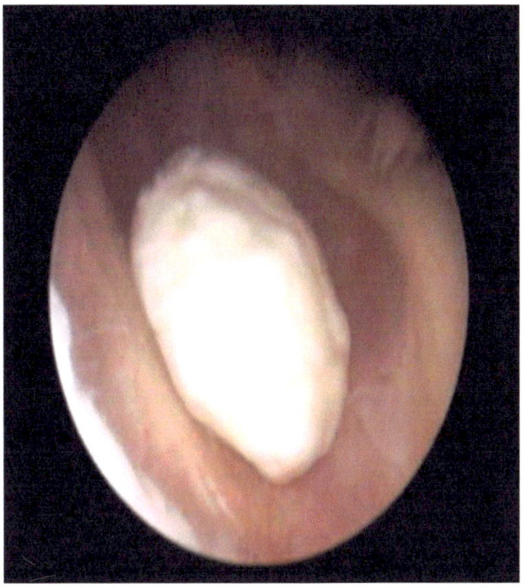

Figure 11.
Recess is often placed where we could find loose bodies.

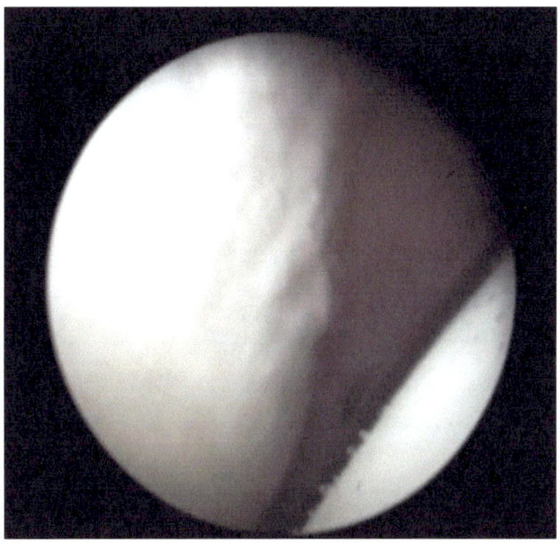

Figure 12.
The cartilage is white, shiny, and smooth. By rotating the optical for 90°, we can see articular surface of the patella, with the same characteristics.

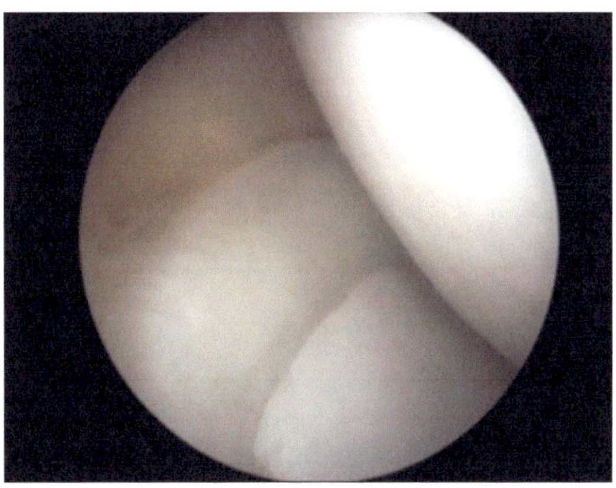

Figure 13.
Healthy meniscus (white, smooth, with sharp inner edge).

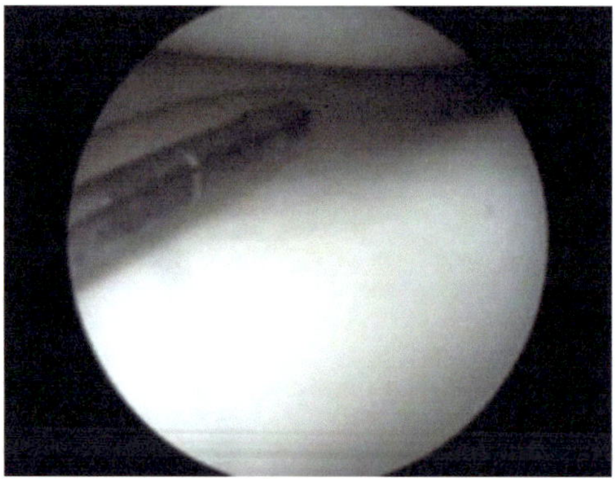

Figure 14.
The attachment of the posterior horn of the medial meniscus.

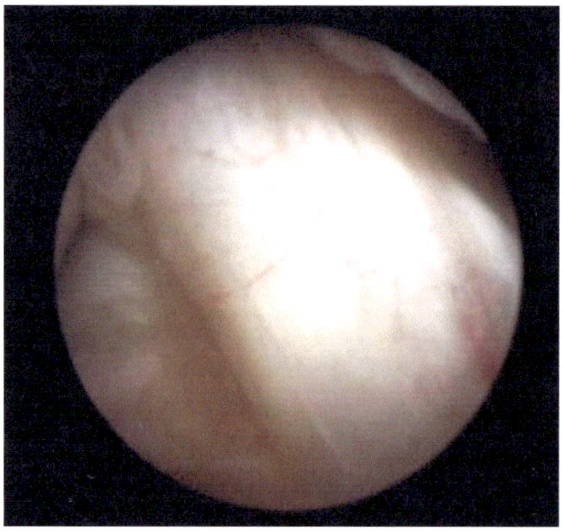

Figure 15.
Course of the ligament (best viewed by flexing the knee).

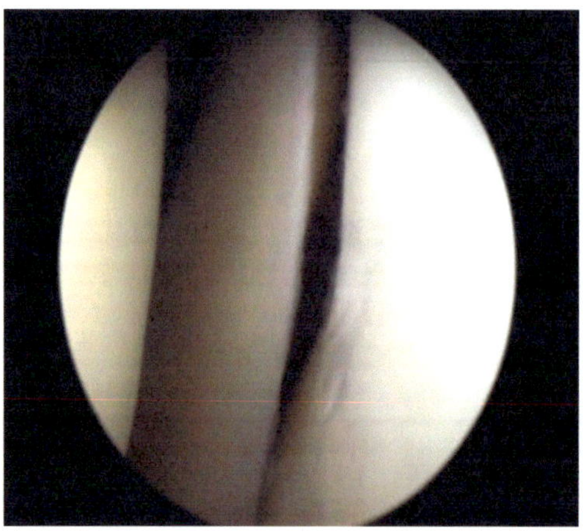

Figure 16.
Lifting up the meniscus, the popliteal tendon is visible in the popliteal aperture.

upward and backward to the attachment on the posterior part of the lateral femoral condyle. The course of the ligament is best viewed by flexing the knee (**Figure 15**). Moving the scope near the central position and pushing it slightly, we can identify the femoral site insertion. PCL is covered by synovial sheet and is not routinely visible until the synovium is removed by a power shaver. Placing the scope beneath ACL and medial femoral condyle and pushing the scope slightly posteriorly, we can identify posterior horn of the medial meniscus and posterior joint capsule. For better visualization the posteromedial portal is used. In the front part, we can see the anterior attachments of both menisci and transvers knee ligament. For examination of the lateral compartment, we must place the knee in the "figure of four" position. Attachments of anterior and posterior horns of the lateral meniscus are near each other. The inner edge is similar to the medial meniscus. In the central third, there is no menisco-capsular junction, and when we lift up the meniscus, the popliteal tendon is visible in the popliteal aperture (**Figure 16**). Ligaments of Wrisberg and Humphry are sometimes visible.

4. Conclusion

Knee arthroscopy is one of the most performed procedures in orthopedic surgery. Nowadays, it is mostly a therapeutic procedure, only in rare cases is diagnostic. Knowing arthroscopic anatomy is essential. The ability to recognize normal shape and appearance of the knee joint structures is the first step in long learning curve for further arthroscopy surgeon.

Author details

Vaso Kecojevic[1]*, Vladimir Harhaji[2] and Srđan Ninković[1]

1 Clinical Center of Vojvodina, Department for Orthopedic Surgery and Traumatology, Novi Sad, Serbia

2 University of Novi Sad, Faculty of Medicine, Novi Sad, Serbia

*Address all correspondence to: keckons@gmail.com

References

[1] Watanabe M, Takada S, Ikeuchi H. Atlas of Arthroscopy. Tokyo: Igaku-Shoin; 1969

[2] Dandy DJ. Arthroscopic Surgery of the Knee. Edinburgh: Churchill Livingstone; 1981

[3] Hunziker EB, Staubli H-U, Jakob RP. Surgical anatomy of the knee joint. In: The Knee and the Cruciate Ligaments. Berlin Heidelberg: Springer-Verlag; 1992. pp. 32-46

[4] Haimes JL, Wroble RR, Grood ES, Noyes FR. Role of the medial structures in the intact and anterior cruciate ligament-deficient knee. Limits of motion in the human knee. The American Journal of Sports Medicine. 1994;**22**:402-409

[5] Greis PE, Bardana DD, Holmstrom MC, et al. Meniscal injury: I. Basic science and evaluation. The Journal of the American Academy of Orthopaedic Surgeons. 2002;**10**:168-176.5

[6] Peters TJ, Smillie IS. Studies on the chemical composition of the menisci of the knee joint with special reference to the horizontal cleavage lesion. Clinical Orthopaedics. 1972;**86**:245-252.48

[7] Mow VC. Structure and function relationships of the meniscus in the knee. In: Mow VC, Arnoczky S, Jackson D, editors. Knee Meniscus: Basic and Clinical Foundations. New York, NY: Raven Press; 1992. pp. 37-58

[8] Simon S. Anatomy, biology, and biomechanics of tendon, ligament, and meniscus. In: Simon S, Wilson J, editors. Orthopaedic Basic Science. Columbus, OH: American Academy of Orthopaedic Surgeons; 1994. p. 54

[9] Arnoczky SP, Warren RF. Microvasculature of the human meniscus. The American Journal of Sports Medicine. 1982;**10**:90-95

[10] Haut RC. The mechanical and viscoelastic properties of the anterior cruciate ligament and af ACL fascicles. In: Jackson DW, Arnoczky SP, Woo SL-Y, Frank CB, Simon TM, editors. The Anterior Cruciate Ligament: Current and Future Concepts. New York: Raven Press; 1993. pp. 63-73

[11] Amis AA, Dawkins GPC. Functional anatomy of the anterior cruciate ligament. Fibre bundle actions related to ligament replacements and injuries. Journal of Bone and Joint Surgery. 1991;**73-B**(2):260-267

[12] Aspden RM, Yarker YE, Hukins WL. Collagen orientations in the meniscus of the knee joint. Journal of Anatomy. 1985;**140**:371-380

[13] Petersen W, Tillmann B. Collagenous fibril texture of the human knee joint menisci. Anatomy and Embryology (Berlin). 1998;**197**:317-324

Section 3

Bioengineering

Chapter 3

Novel Approaches in Meniscal Repair Utilizing Mesenchymal Stem Cells, New Generation Bioscaffolds and Biological Adhesives as Cell Delivery Vehicles

James Melrose

Abstract

Mesenchymal stem cells (MSCs) have been widely applied in the repair of the knee-joint menisci which have a limited ability to undergo spontaneous repair. The menisci stabilise the knee-joint and are weight-bearing structures subjected to considerable tensional and compressive forces during flexion-extension and torsional loading of the knee. Traumatic loading of the knee-joint menisci can generate a number of lesions in the inner avascular meniscal regions. These have a limited capability of intrinsic repair and predispose the underlying articular cartilages to premature osteoarthritis. A number of strategies have therefore been developed for meniscal repair employing MSCs, bioscaffolds, hydrogels, biological glue cell delivery systems and agents which promote cell proliferation/matrix synthesis. Meniscal implants have also been developed in combination with the above procedures. It is important that meniscal defects be repaired not only to maintain knee-joint stability but also to prevent further degenerative changes in other knee joint tissues. Degenerative menisci contribute degradative proteinases and inflammatory mediators to the total synovial degradative proteinase pool. Partial or total surgical removal of the menisci is not a solution since this leads to premature osteoarthritis. Meniscal integrity needs to be maintained or repair strategies implemented in a timely manner to maintain knee joint function.

Keywords: meniscal repair, mesenchymal stem cell, bioscaffolds, biological glues, meniscal implants/allografts

1. Introduction

1.1 Meniscal structure: function

The knee joint menisci provide joint stability during weight bearing, the curved superior meniscal surfaces provide congruity between the curved femoral condyle and flat tibial articular cartilages [1]. The menisci act as shock absorbers and protect

IntechOpen

the weight bearing articular tissues from excessive point loading [2] transferring forces between the femoral and tibial joint surfaces, transmitting 50–90% of the total knee joint load during weight-bearing [3, 4]. The structural organisation of the meniscus is designed to withstand circumferential hoop stresses which are generated within the meniscal tissue to dissipate tensile stresses which are transferred along the circumferential meniscal collagen fibre networks counteracting the tendency of the menisci to be extruded peripherally when the knee joint is subjected to compressive loading [5]. Energy is absorbed into the collagen fibres by the dynamic expulsion of joint fluid from the aggrecan-hyaluronan macro-aggregate networks entrapped within the meniscal collagenous networks. The menisci are fibre reinforced structures stiffening and protecting them from damage by excessive deformation during compressive loading [6] (**Figure 1a** and **b**).

The contribution of intact menisci in knee load-bearing is emphasised from the increase in contact forces in the underlying articular cartilages of up to 350% following partial or total meniscectomy where as little as 16–34% of the intact meniscus may be removed [1, 3, 7]. Radial meniscal tears which extend to its periphery may result in significant contact forces being transmitted to the underlying articular cartilages which can damage these tissues [8].

Water (~70% wet weight) and collagen, (mainly type I, and lower amounts of type II, III and VI collagen constitute 60–70% of the meniscal dry weight) are major meniscal components [9–15]. Proteoglycans (aggrecan, decorin, biglycan, versican, fibromodulin, lumican, keratocan) and elastic microfibrillar glycoproteins are quantitatively minor meniscal extracellular matrix (ECM) components but convey essential functional properties [14–16]. The meniscus is a complex fibre-reinforced structure designed to withstand multidirectional tensional and compressive forces (**Figure 1a** and **b**). The outer third of the meniscus (red zone) is served by a fine capillary network. Defects in this region of the meniscus have the ability to undergo spontaneous repair however the inner two thirds of the meniscus (white zone) is avascular and has a limited ability to undergo repair (**Figure 2a**). The outer zone of the meniscus is a collagen rich fibrocartilaginous tissue while the inner zone contains higher proteoglycan levels and is cartilaginous (**Figure 2b**). Immunolocalisation of perlecan, HSPG2, a large modular HS multifunctional proteoglycan demonstrates a strong localisation pattern in this inner region. Perlecan is marker of chondrogenesis [17–20].

Supraphysiological overload of the menisci may generate defects in the inner meniscus diminishing its weight bearing capability and ability to resist tensional stresses and it becomes less able to dissipate such forces to prevent overloading of the underlying articular cartilage. A number of characteristic tears (bucket-handle, degenerate) occur in the inner meniscal region. Longitudinal and radial tears can also affect the outer meniscus (**Figure 2c**). This can also damage the underlying articular cartilages formerly protected by the menisci leading to degenerative changes and impacting on the knee's ability to act efficiently as an articulating weight bearing structure. Development of premature osteoarthritis (OA) may also result in such circumstances [21, 22]. Menisci in OA knees are also subject to ectopic focal depositions of calcium in cyst like structures (**Figure 2d**). Fibrillation of the inner meniscal region is also a common degenerative feature in OA. Meniscal cell clustering adjacent to such fibrillations is also common and may indicate endogenous adult stem cell activity in response to altered biomechanics/nutrition in this region. Cell clustering has also been observed adjacent to surface fibrillations in OA articular cartilage and adjacent to lesions in the annulus fibrosus of the degenerate intervertebral disc [23–29]. Such cell clustering may be indicative of an incomplete frustrated repair response by resident adult stem cells.

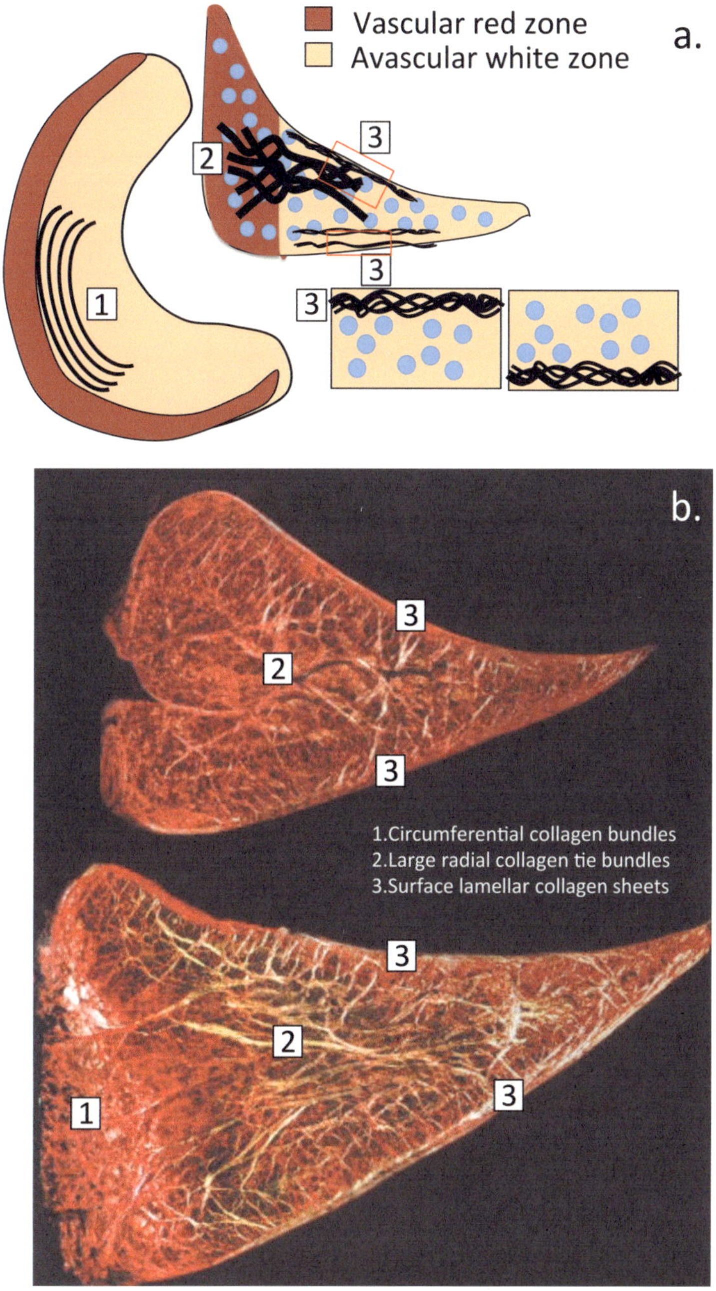

Figure 1.
Diagrammatic representation of the collagenous organisation in a meniscus. (i) The meniscus contains a complex arrangement of radial collagen fibre bundles in the outer meniscus, (ii) thick radial tie bundles internally as well as (iii) finer collagen fibre bundles of collagen in lamellar sheets in the inferior and superior meniscal surfaces. Notice that the inferior lamina is significantly thicker than the superior lamina. Vertical radial sections through 2 year old lateral and medial ovine menisci stained with picrosirius red and viewed under polarised light depicting collagen bundles which are highly refractile due to their ordered collagenous structure appearing as bright rod-like structures (b). Picrosirius red predominantly visualises the major fibrillar meniscal collagen, type I collagen. Methodology for Picrosirius red staining is as described earlier [78].

Many strategies have consequently been developed to effect meniscal repair using a number of cell types including mesenchymal stem cells (MSCs) sourced from a number of tissues (**Table 1**), and combinations of bioscaffolds, hydrogels,

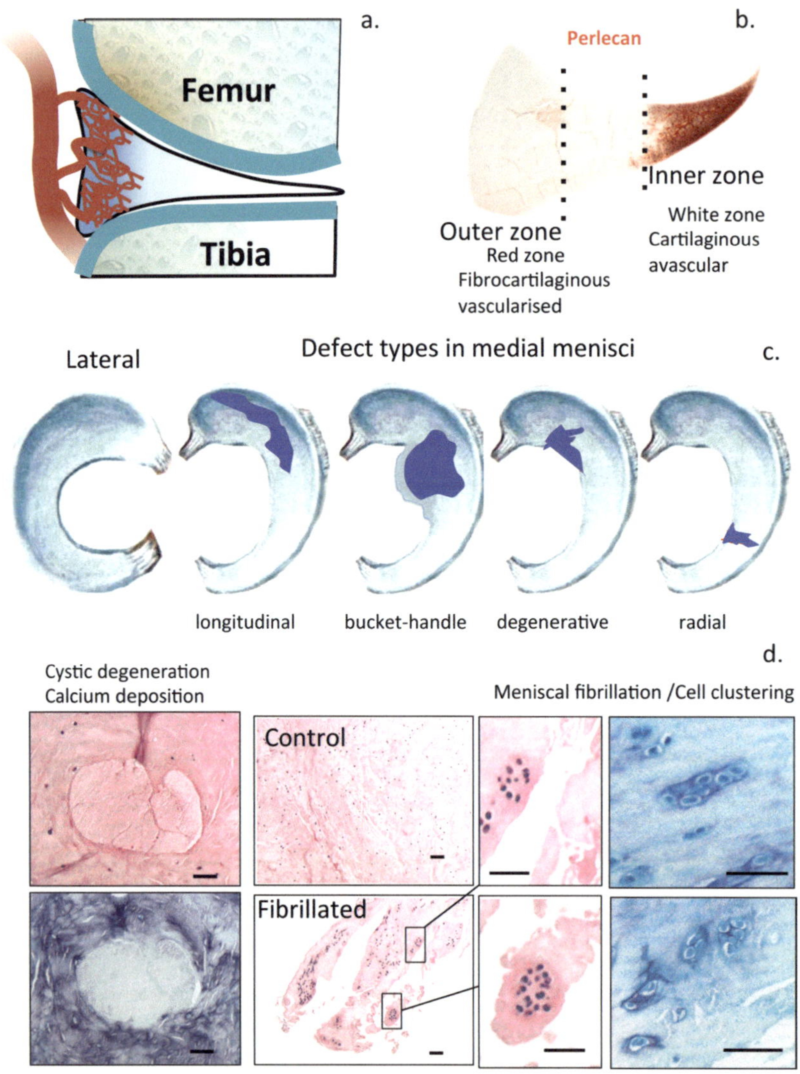

Figure 2.
Structural features evident in the normal and degenerate meniscus. Diagrammatic representation of the vascularisation of a vertically sectioned meniscus showing the extensive capillary network in the outer meniscal red zone and lack of a blood supply to the inner two thirds of the meniscus (a). The inner meniscus is a cartilage like tissue which is well delineated in a newborn meniscus by immunolocalisation of perlecan, HSPG2, a chondrogenic marker proteoglycan (b). Menisci are subject to a number of structural defects which are summarised diagrammatically (c). Histochemical visualisation (H & E) and toluidine blue staining, of some features of degenerate menisci (d). Focal deposition of small calcium deposits in a cyst like formation in the outer meniscus zone in a 53 year old human meniscus. Fibrillation of the inner meniscal zone and cell cluster formation. In the normal meniscus single cells are distributed throughout the meniscus with no clustering.

bioadhesive cell delivery systems and bioactive agents which stimulate the resident and exogenous cells applied for therapeutic purposes (**Tables 2** and **3**).

In-vitro experiments have shown that co-culture of bone marrow derived stromal stem cells with meniscal cells increases cell proliferation and matrix synthesis [30]. Type I and type II collagen and aggrecan mRNA expression were elevated and ECM protein levels increased (**Figure 3a** and **b**). Significantly, meniscal cells stimulated with FGF-2 or FGF-18 in 3D pellet culture also produced elevated levels of these ECM components (**Figure 3c** and **d**). MSCs are believed to act both through transfer of material directly to resident cell populations through cell-cell contact

MSC source	Lesion or study type	References
Intra-articular injection synovial MSCs	Avascular tear	[143]
Rabbit meniscal MSCs	Central meniscal defect	[155]
Synovium derived MSCs	Longitudinal tears and punch holes	[142, 144, 145]
Targeted intra-articularly delivered super-paramagnetic FeO labelled adipose MSCs	Massive lesions encompassing the avascular zone	[146]
Bone marrow, adipose, synovium, meniscus derived MSC delivery to tears in fibrin glue/gel/clot, scaffold	Literature Review of MSCs used in meniscal repair in multiple animal models	[44, 45]
Bone marrow and meniscal derived MSCs	In vitro cell culture	[148]
Blood vessel derived MSCs	Avascular tears	[151]
Bone marrow derived MSCs and fibrin glue	Closure of meniscal tears	[149]
Collagen membrane wrapped meniscal defects injected with MSCs	Tears in avascular zone	[156]
Co-cultured synovial stem cell-meniscal cell cultures	In-vitro demonstration of superior cell proliferation with co-culture compared to monoculture	[43]
Systematic review of the use of MSCs in meniscal repair	Promising results in human meniscal repair	[152]
Comparison of autologous MSCs and meniscal cells for meniscal repair	Rabbit meniscal model punch defect, successful repair of meniscal defects in OARSI grade 3.1 early OA tissues by both cell types	[46–48]
hMSCs delivery in a decellularized ECM to meniscal defects in a nude rat model	Delivery system appropriate for repair purposes	[158]
Review of hMSCs in human meniscal repair	Autologous adipose tissue-derived stem cells or culture-expanded bone marrow-derived stem cells were both suitable for meniscal repair	[153]
Prospective, open-label first-in-human safety clinical trial of hMSCs delivered in collagen scaffold in patients with an avascular meniscal tear	Repair of torn avascular meniscal cartilage by undifferentiated hMSCs harvested from iliac crest bone marrow biopsy. Significant clinical improvement over 2 years, no recurrence of meniscal tears	[157]
3D co-culture meniscal cell: equine MSCs in collagen type I tissue derived small intestinal ECM bioscaffold	Favourable in-vitro results obtained with cells of meniscal cellular morphology attained by MSCs and expression of type I, II collagen	[160]
Allogeneic adipose derived stem cells in scaffold free tissue engineered construct	Rabbit model using 1.5 mm circular defects in anterior horn of medial menisci filled with MSCs in bioscaffold gave positive results	[147]
A review of cell based approaches in meniscal repair	An assessment of mono and co-culture approaches with meniscal cells and MSCs in bioscaffolds and scaffold free approaches	[154]
3D MSC: meniscal fibrochondrocyte co-cultures for meniscal repair	Change in MSC morphology to a fibrochondrocytic phenotype is conducive to meniscal repair	[159]

Table 1.
Mesenchymal stem cell (MSC) sources used in therapeutic approaches for meniscal repair.

Method/polymer	Details of technique	References
Regen Menaflex™ collagen meniscal implant	Resorbable meniscal implant, however the FDA removed approval for device in 2013	[87]
Actifit synthetic meniscal substitute to stabilise knee	Post meniscectomy allogeneic implant with cell infiltration into implant from meniscal wall	[88]
Medial meniscus allograft transplantation (MAT) using a modified bone plug	Meniscal allograft harvested using an arthroscopic bone plug technique	[100]
Anatomically shaped polycarbonate-urethane meniscal implant	Artificial meniscal implant designed for the preservation of articular cartilage	[93]
Polycarbonate-urethane implant	Meniscal replacement	[91]
Thermoplastic polyurethane implant	Meniscal replacement	[98, 219]
Salt modified crosslinked PVA hydrogel meniscus cell implant	Meniscal shaped flexible implants for meniscal replacement	[95]
Polycaprolactone supplemented with slow release microbeads containing CTGF and TGF-$\beta 3$	3D printed meniscus	[103, 106]
Interpenetrating network gels of poly(2-acrylamido-2-methylpropanesulfonate) and polyacrylamide	3D printed meniscal replacement	[104]

Table 2.
Meniscal allografts and implants used for meniscal repair and replacement.

Scaffolds	Lesion and study type	References
Myoblast loaded PLGA mesh scaffold	Avascular tears	[172]
HYADD4® HA hydrogel cell delivery	Radial-longitudinal tears	[173]
Electro spun type I collagen scaffolds and vascular/avascular region meniscal cells	Avascular meniscal tears	[174]
Radio opaque electro spun scaffold	Meniscal regrowth	[176]
Wrapping of meniscal defects with collagen membrane and injection of MSCs	Tears in avascular zone	[156]
Aligned electro spun nano fibrous scaffold	Radial tear	[178]
Collagen gel scaffold or HA hydrogel delivery of meniscal, synovial and adipose cells	Bucket handle tear	[177]
Type I collagen scaffold/ infrapatellar fat pad	Anterior 2 mm round holes	[179]
Chondrocyte + PLGA mesh scaffold + PRP	Chondrocytes evaluated	[180]
Meniscal cells in fibre reinforced collagen-GAG scaffold + PRP	Gene profiling study	[168]

Scaffolds	Lesion and study type	References
Juvenile meniscus fragments	Avascular tears	[181]
A review of biomaterials used in meniscal repair	An assessment of state of the art materials currently in use in meniscal repair	[197]
Tissue derived ECM scaffolds	Biological scaffolds derived from cell and tissue-derived ECM have shown great promise in tissue engineering maintaining the biological and biomechanical properties, structure, and function of the native meniscus	[198]
A comprehensive review of hydrogels used in meniscal repair	A number of hydrogels exhibiting high water regain provide a 3D microenvironment with variable topographical properties typical of meniscal tissue and useful platforms for cellular colonisation. Controlled delivery of bioactive molecules has been built into the design of some of these scaffolds to enhance repair processes	[200]
Decellularised, micronized ECM scaffolds for improved meniscal repair	Decellularised menisci cryoground into a powder was cytocompatible with meniscal fibrochondrocytes, synoviocytes. Cellular infiltration and proliferation demonstrated the ability of this scaffold to promote cellular survival, migration, and proliferation and meniscal repair	[198]
Rapidly dissociation of autologous meniscal cells enhances their healing properties	Bovine meniscal cells were isolated by rapid dissociation using collagenase and applied in a fibrin gel to a radial meniscal tear. This procedure enhanced the healing properties of the seeded cells inserted into the meniscal defect	[199]
Bioactive supplements added to scaffolds		
Multiple injection of leukoreduced PRP	ACL and meniscal repair	[165]
10% human serum, 5% PRP, 5% autologous plasma	Non-vascular meniscal lesions	[166]
Human chondrocyte-seeded PLGA scaffold + PRP	Testing of biocompatibility of bio scaffold in nude mice	[170, 197]
PRP plasma for anterior cruciate ligament and meniscal repair	A review of clinical and basic science strategies aimed at biological augmentation of the healing response	[120]
Platelet-rich plasma for open meniscal repair in young patients	Effective treatment of horizontal tears extending into the avascular zone	[171]
Platelet-rich fibrin for meniscal repair	PRP-fibrin promotes rabbit meniscus repair by meniscocyte Proliferation, migration, and ECM synthesis	[220]
Fibrin clot augmentation	Fibrin clot augments meniscal repair	[221]
Platelet rich fibrin clot	Repair of horizontal meniscal defects	[222]
Platelet rich plasma for meniscal repair	Prospective, randomized, double-blind, placebo-controlled study evaluating healing of unstable complete vertical bucket handle meniscal healing, of unstable, complete vertical meniscal tears (Bucket Handle)	[169]

Scaffolds	Lesion and study type	References
Administration of an EGF inhibitor in a customised collagen bio scaffold	Meniscal regeneration in a rabbit model	[223]
Administration of Simvastin in meniscal repair	Repair of avascular defects in a rabbit meniscal defect model	[224]
Overexpression of TGF-β via rAAV-mediated gene transfer	Healing of human meniscal lesions	[183]
rAAV overexpression of TGF-β	Complex meniscal tears	[183]
Transduced IGF-1 over-expressing meniscal cells	Avascular tears	[184]
Liposome gene transfer IGF-1 meniscal cells	Avascular tears	[185]
Chondrocyte, VEGF, BMP-7, matrigel, HA cultures	Inner avascular tears	[186]
Intra-articular injection of microRNA-210	Avascular tears	[187]
Fibrin-CTGF stimulates meniscal cell to repair inner zone meniscal defects	Avascular tears	[188]
Serum, HA, TGF-β3 supplemented scaffold directed repair of meniscal tears	Directed repair of meniscal tears	[182]
Non-viral gene transfer to meniscal cells and FGF-2 overexpressing meniscal cells	FGF-2 transduced meniscal cells in alginate beads	[190, 191]
VEGF stimulation of resident meniscal cells	Avascular tears	[194]
TGF-β1 induction of meniscal cell proliferation and migration to a meniscal defect	Micro wound assay system	[195]
OP-1 putty in punch biopsy meniscal holes	2 mm holes—inner meniscus	[196]
Gelatin hydrogel + FGF-2	Horizontal tears	[192]
HA-collagen composite + PRP	2 mm holes, implant	[47, 193]
Type I collagen scaffold and infrapatellar fat pad	Repair of 2mm meniscal defects	[179]
Intra-articular injection of micro RNA 210	Promotes angiogenesis and repair of avascular meniscal defects	[187]
Use of BMP-7 for meniscal repair	healing of circular defects in avascular region by OP-1 putty	[186]
VEGF, BMP-7, Matrigel™, hyaluronic acid, in vitro cultured chondrocytes for meniscal repair	Healing of defects in the inner two thirds of the meniscus	[186]
Electro spun gelatin/poly(lactic acid-co-glycolic acid) bilayered nanofiber scaffolds for meniscal repair	PLGA nanofibre reinforced scaffolds have useful properties and are compatible as a substrate for meniscal repair	[175]

Scaffolds	Lesion and study type	References
HYADD4 based hydrogel for meniscal repair	Intra-articular administration of HYADD4 hydrogel to human knees containing degenerative meniscal tears improved VAS pain clinical indices and improved knee functionality based on WOMAC scores	[173]
Electro spun collagen bio scaffolds for meniscal repair	Electro spun collagen type I scaffolds seeded with human meniscal cells placed in longitudinal avascular meniscal defects stimulated meniscal repair as assessed by histology, immunohistochemistry, mechanical testing, and MRI	[174]
Aligned electro spun nano fibrous scaffolds for meniscal repair	Repair of meniscal radial tears using aligned electro spun Nano fibrous scaffolds seeded with meniscal fibrochondrocytes	[178]
Non-viral gene transfer systems of possible application in meniscal repair	A comparison of 18 non-viral gene transfer systems to identify an efficient transfection system for primary cultures of juvenile and adult human meniscal fibrochondrocytes. Overexpression of FGF-2 following transfection with FGF-2 increased meniscal fibrochondrocyte proliferation but not GAG synthesis	[190, 191]
Bio adhesives		
Pre-treatment of meniscal surfaces with collagenase and TGF-β3 prior to use of bio adhesives for meniscal repair	Enzymatic pre-treatment improves effectiveness of bio adhesives	[225]
Biodegradable hyper-branched adhesives for meniscal repair	Sealing of meniscal tears	[211]
CS-bone marrow tissue adhesive	Novel bone marrow derived CS adhesive suitable for securing repair tissue interfaces	[214]
3D PGA-HA bio scaffold stabilized with fibrin	ECM repair by meniscal cells	[189]
New generation meniscal adhesives	Inner avascular lesions	[211]
Re-attachment of horizontal meniscal tears	Fibrin re-attachment	[215]
Mussel based bio adhesives	bio adhesives containing bactericidal and fundgicidal activity and improved wet strength for reattachment of surgical incisions	[216, 217]

Abbreviations: PRP, platelet rich plasma; rAAV, recombinant Adeno-Associated Virus; PGA, polyglycolic acid; HYADD4®, hyaluronan derivative; PLGA, polylactic-co-glycolic acid, CTGF, connective tissue growth factor; VEGF, vascular endothelial cell growth factor; OP-1, osteogenic protein-1; CS, chondroitin sulphate; FGF-2, fibroblast growth factor-2; TGF-β, transforming growth factor-β.

Table 3.
Meniscal repair using bio scaffolds, bioactive substances and bio adhesives.

and also by secretion of trophic factors which both stimulate tissue regenerative processes [31–42]. Co-cultures of synovial stem cells [43] and MSCs [44–48] with meniscal cells have been evaluated in a number of biomatrices for meniscal repair purposes (**Table 1**).

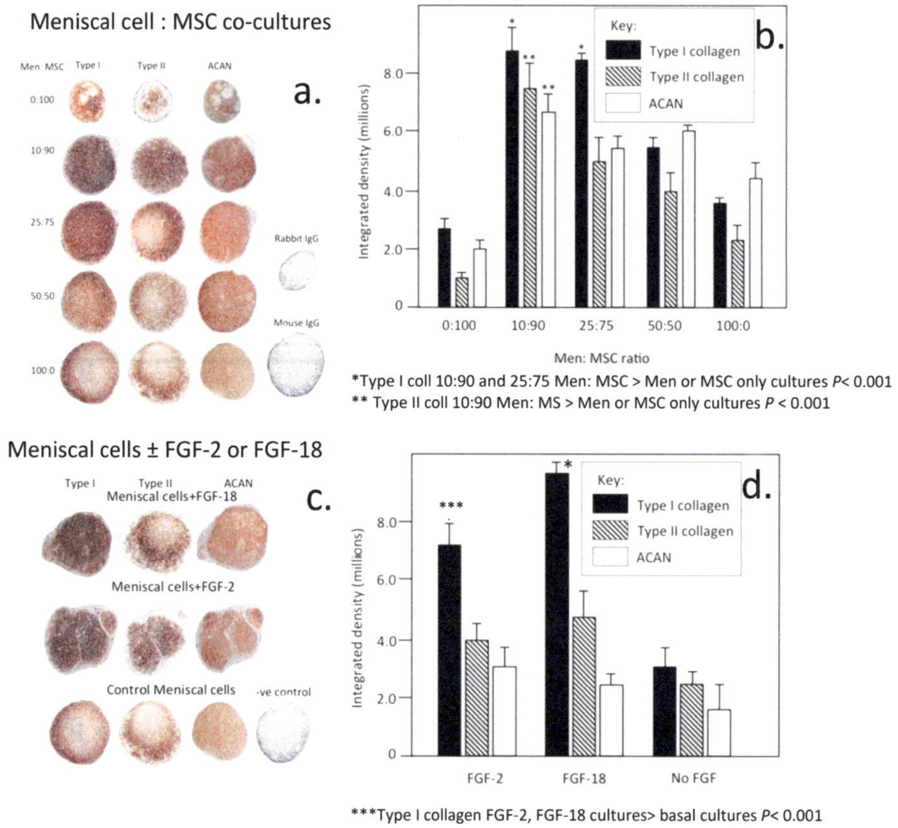

Figure 3.
Co-culture of meniscal cells and bone marrow derived mesenchymal stromal cells induces cell proliferation and ECM production and is recapitulated to some degree by treatment of meniscal cells with FGF-2 and FGF-18. Immunolocalisation of meniscal matrix components in micro-mass pellet culture. Immunolocalisation of type I collagen, type II collagen and aggrecan (ACAN) in meniscal-MSC micro-mass pellet co-cultures (a). Negative controls of pellets using rabbit IgG (MSC pellet) and mouse IgG (meniscal cell pellet) for immunolocalisation in the absence of primary antibody. Anti-type I collagen (clone I-8H5) and anti-type II collagen (clone II-4CII) were from MP Biomedicals, Ohio, USA. A rabbit polyclonal antibody (pAb) # 2194 to aggrecan G1 domain was a gift from Dr. J Mort Joint Diseases laboratory, Shriners, Hospital for Children, McGill University, Montreal, QC, Canada [218]. PAb 2194 was raised against a mixture of four aggrecan specific G1 peptide-ovalbumin conjugates including HDNSLSVSIPQPSGGC, RVLLGTSLTIPCYFIDPMHPVTTAPS, TEGRVRVNSAYQDKGGC and SSRYDAICYTG (single letter amino acid code). Morphometric image analysis of meniscal matrix components produced in pellet culture. Quantitation of type I and type II collagen and aggrecan immunolocalisation levels in meniscal: MSC co-cultures using Adobe Photoshop CS4 morphometric image analysis software as integrated pixel density. Mean values ± SD for 3 pellet sections is shown (b). Immunolocalisation of matrix components produced by meniscal cells in pellet cultures stimulated with FGF-2 and FGF-18. Immunolocalisation of Type I and Type II collagen and aggrecan (ACAN) in meniscal cell micromass pellet cultures stimulated with FGF-2 and FGF-18 (a–c) for 21 days (c). Morphometric image analysis of meniscal matrix components using Adobe Photoshop CS4 morphometric image analysis software (d).

2. Meniscus preserving therapies

2.1 Why it is important to preserve the knee joint meniscus? A historical perspective

The meniscus was historically considered a vestigial muscle remnant and little importance was attributed to this structure for knee joint function. Consequently, radical surgery and total removal of the meniscus were common surgical practice in the 1980s with serious long-term consequences for the meniscectomised knee. It should have been obvious from meniscectomy studies used to induce OA experimentally in animals that surgical removal of the menisci from knee joints was not a benign procedure [49–74]. However it took time for these animal findings to be translated to human studies [59–61, 65, 67, 70, 72] and for these experimental findings to be fed through to human clinical practice and the importance of the meniscus in entirety in knee joint articulation, weight bearing and load distribution became established. Even so, publications were still appearing as late as 2016 emphasising the importance of the preservation of the knee joint menisci to ensure optimal knee joint function three decades after meniscal removal had been shown to induce degenerative changes in other knee joint tissues [75].

Currently, the consensus in the surgical treatment of meniscal tears is to preserve as much functional meniscal tissue as possible to preserve knee joint function [76].

The menisci play critical protective roles for the knee joint articular cartilages through shock absorption and load distribution and also have important roles to play in proprioception and balance [5]. The ESSKA (European Society for Sports Traumatology, Knee Surgery and Arthroscopy) MENISCUS CONSENSUS INITIATIVE was initiated in 2014 to find a European consensus on the treatment of meniscus pathologies [76].

Further studies in animals [73, 77–79] established a more direct contribution from meniscal degeneration to joint structures globally during degenerative conditions such as OA and RA. During the development of arthritic conditions in animals [73, 77, 79] and humans [80] tissue proteoglycans become fragmented through proteolytic degradation and this reduces the weight bearing and articulatory properties of the articular cartilages and menisci and may even impact on subchondral bone [80]. Matrix metalloproteases (MMPs), ADAMTS (A Disintegrin and Metalloproteinase with Thrombospondin motifs)-4 and ADAMTS-5 produced by articular chondrocytes have a major impact on aggrecan and other cartilage proteoglycans reducing the weight bearing properties of the knee joint articular cartilages. The increase in synovial degradative protease pool during OA and RA was previously attributed to the articular chondrocytes which respond to inflammatory cytokines in the arthritic joint by producing these degradative proteases. Recent in-vitro studies have however now shown that meniscal fibrochondrocytes also potently respond to interleukin-1 and tumour necrosis factor-α by producing significant levels of MMPs (MMP-1, 2, 3, 9, 13), ADAMTS-4 and ADAMTS-5 and are a major cellular source of these components in the total global degradative enzyme pool present in synovial fluid [81–83]. Meniscal cells actually produce higher levels of these degradative components than articular chondrocytes, thus represent a previously unidentified therapeutic target in the treatment of OA and RA.

2.2 Meniscal implants

Partial or total meniscal replacement by collagen or synthetic allografts following meniscectomy have yielded mixed results (**Table 2**) [84, 85]. Implants fall into two categories, (i) porous, resorbable implants which stimulate tissue regeneration and (ii) solid, non-resorbable implants which physically replace the meniscus [86]. The Regen Menaflex™ collagen total meniscal implant (CMI®, Ivy Sports Medicine) is a resorbable implant. A review of the CMI® by Hansen et al. in a 10 year follow up confirmed good clinical outcomes, solid integration of the CMI® with host tissue and it was concluded that the CMI® held promise for meniscal repair [87]. After a protracted series of re-reviews of experimental data, technical issues and protocols the FDA rescinded approval for the Menaflex® device in 2013. The Actifit® polymeric polyurethane partial implant (ORTEQ Sports Medicine) is a honeycomb scaffold that enables blood-flow through it providing a route for cellular in-growth as the body's natural healing process takes place. Once the damaged section of the meniscus surgically removed the implant is attached to an area of the remaining meniscus with a good blood supply [86]. This has improved knee joint function and reduced knee pain in patients for up to 5 years after implantation and a stable cartilage profile was achieved in 46.7% of patients but a relatively high failure rate was also reported [88–90].

An artificial Polycarbonate-urethane implant has been developed for replacement of the medial meniscus [91–93]. NUsurface® have developed a polyethylene reinforced polycarbonate urethane total meniscal implant, approved for use in Europe since 2008 and in Israel since 2011 [94]. The safety and long-term performance of the NUsurface implant is currently under evaluation in SUN (Safety Using NUsurface®) and VENUS (Verifying the Effectiveness of the NUsurface® System) clinical trials in the USA.

Salt modified cross-linked PVA based hydrogels seeded with meniscal cells have been evaluated for meniscal repair [95] as have polyglycolic acid implants seeded with chondrocytes [96] and (poly-(3-hydroxybutyrate-co-3-hydroxyvalerate) meniscal implants seeded with fibrochondrocytes [97].

Biodegradable thermoplastic polyurethane Estane® polymer (Lubrizol Corp, USA) porous implants have been evaluated in dogs as a meniscal replacement [98]. Colonisation of the implant by resident meniscal synovial cells from the peripheral attachments, laying down of matrix components within the implant and the biointegration of the implant to the peripheral meniscal attachment tissues were evaluated 3–6 month post implantation. This demonstrated that the implant filled completely with meniscal tissue as demonstrated by toluidine blue staining for proteoglycan, and for type II collagen and I by immunolocalisations using specific collagen antibodies. Histological evaluation of the tibia and femoral articular cartilages confirmed these tissues did not degenerate in the experimental period employed for this study.

A number of critical reviews on the performance of meniscal implants [86, 87, 99–101] generally acknowledge that despite initial promising findings long-term and randomised controlled studies still need to be undertaken to confirm implant performance and reliability for meniscal repair and that the development of a meniscal replacement tissue of comparable performance to native tissue has yet to be achieved.

2.3 3D printing of knee joint menisci

Polycaprolactone has been used as a scaffolding material to form an exact meniscal replica using a 3D printer [102–105]. MRI scans of the meniscus are converted into a 3D image, data from this image is then used to drive a 3D printer, which produces a scaffold in the exact shape of the meniscus, down to a resolution of 10 μm. Differential release of CTGF and TGF-β3 to drive formation initially of the outer collagenous meniscal region then the more cartilaginous inner meniscus is achieved by slow release microspheres containing CTGF and TGF-β3 in the printed meniscus. These attract meniscal progenitor cells into the scaffold which lay down tissue gradients to form the collagenous outer and cartilaginous inner regions of the meniscus. In sheep this takes between 4 and 6 weeks to achieve meniscal replacement and the scaffolding material then slowly redissolves to be eliminated by normal resorptive processes.

Interpenetrating networks of poly(2-acrylamido-2-methylpropanesulfonate) and polyacrylamide can be prepared by varying the ratio of polyacrylamide to cross-linker, to yield a gel with compression strength and elastic modulus of 61.9 and 0.44 MPa. This gel has maximum compressive and tensile strengths of 93.5 and 1.4 MPa respectively. This can be used in a 3D printer to prepare replacement menisci from a patients X-ray computed tomography image of a meniscus [104]. Slow release of CTGF and TGF-β3 from a 3D printed meniscus stimulated endogenous stem/progenitor cells to undertake meniscal regeneration [106].

3. Meniscus regenerative therapies

3.1 Therapeutic use of mesenchymal stem cells in tissue repair

Mesenchymal stem cells (MSCs) have been the subject of intense investigation since their discovery in the 1960s due to their remarkable efficacy in tissue repair. MSCs were originally considered to migrate into sites of injury, where they engrafted, and differentiated into functional cells, resulting in regeneration of damaged or diseased connective tissue [107]. Findings from several hundred animal studies and many human clinical trials have challenged this mode of action. MSCs certainly exhibit a remarkable ability to repair diseased tissues, but it has become increasingly apparent that they do not engraft in enough numbers or for sufficient durations in tissue defects to provide tissue repair and clinical benefit directly. Additional modes of action for MSCs have therefore been proposed based on their ability to enhance resident cell viability and/or proliferation, reduce cell apoptosis [108, 109], and, in some cases, modulate immune responses [110–114]. These are due to paracrine effects due to secreted growth factors, cytokines, and hormones by the MSCs and cell-cell interactions mediated through communicating nanotubes, which convey extracellular vesicles containing reparative peptides/proteins, mRNA, and microRNAs [107]. Caplan (2017) has proposed that stem cells should be renamed *Medicinal Signalling Cells* to more accurately reflect how they home in on injured or diseased tissue sites secreting bioactive factors with immunomodulatory and trophic properties which direct the resident cells to undertake the tissue repair process, this may happen long after the MSCs have disappeared from the defect site [115].

MSCs have gained popularity for tissue repair with good reason [32, 116], and several applications have been developed for their use in the repair of connective tissues including the meniscus [117–125].

3.1.1 How do MSCs effect tissue repair?

Despite their widespread use in therapeutic applications the precise mode of action of MSCs remains elusive [126–130]. MSCs undergo engraftment in a defect site and differentiate to an appropriate cell lineage conducive to tissue repair [131] where they act as in-situ reservoirs of trophic factors [132] which direct resident cell populations to effect tissue repair [33, 40, 133–135]. It is un-resolved whether cell-cell contact is essential for MSC action in tissue repair [33, 117, 131]. The pluripotency of MSCs facilitates the differentiation of the engrafted cells to effect tissue repair [33, 133]. However, some evidence shows that only a small proportion of the MSCs actually integrate and survive in the host tissues and the predominant mechanism by which MSCs participate in tissue repair appears to reside in their paracrine activity through the production of a multitude of growth factors and cytokines [33, 132]. Lipid micro vesicles released by MSCs have also been shown to be an important means of cellular communication and occurs alongside the mediators secreted by the MSCs. Nano vesicles/exosomes transfer proteins, lipids and small RNAs to neighbouring cells, and through these mediate a variety of biological responses in addition to those mediated by soluble trophic factors supplied by the MSCs [35, 136, 137].

3.2 Use of MSCs and chondrocytes for meniscal repair

The use of meniscal, chondrocytes or MSCs [138] in tissue engineering [139] using synthetic and biological scaffolds [101] containing bioactive factors [140] hold promise in the repair of the meniscus. Direct intra-synovial injections of MSCs have also been employed and meniscal regeneration and resolution of pain recorded [135, 141]. MSCs sourced from a number of tissues including synovial tissues [142–145], adipose [146, 147], bone marrow [45, 148–150] and blood vessels [151] have been applied in a number of applications to promote meniscal repair [44–48, 152–158] (**Table 1**). Co-cultures of meniscal cells and MSCs have also been examined in meniscal repair strategies [43, 159, 160]. Furthermore, a diverse range of bio scaffolds have been developed containing CS have been developed to promote MSC differentiation in-vivo for varied applications in repair biology [161] (**Table 3**). These scaffolds are also appropriate for strategies aimed at meniscal repair but have yet to be applied in this area.

3.3 Co-culture of MSCs/meniscal cells and in-vitro stimulation with FGF-2/FGF-18

MSCs hold tremendous promise in regenerative medicine however their mode of action remains to be precisely established. Direct cell-cell transfer of stem cell material to resident cells has been shown to promote tissue repair processes, while soluble trophic factors secreted by the stem cells can also stimulate repair. In order to examine these possibilities further in the meniscus, bone marrow MSCs and meniscal cells have been co-cultured in micro-mass pellet cultures (**Figure 3a** and **b**). The influence of FGF-2 and FGF-18 on meniscal pellet cultures have also been assessed to mimic the action of soluble trophic factors (**Figure 3c** and **d**). Immunolocalisation of the extracellular matrix (ECM) components type I and II collagen and aggrecan (ACAN) have been used to assess the response of the meniscal cells to these treatments. Meniscal cell proliferation is significantly elevated by MSC co-culture, and deposition of type I collagen and type II collagen and ACAN elevated. FGF-2 and FGF-18 also increase these ECM components in pellet culture. Cross-talk between meniscal cells and MSCs (and FGF-2 and FGF-18 to a lesser extent) thus positively influence cell proliferation and matrix production conducive to tissue replenishment and repair which would be expected to be re-capitulated in-vivo upon administration of stem cells to meniscal defects. Thus direct cell-cell contact and soluble trophic factors both stimulate meniscal repair processes.

3.4 Bioscaffolds, bioactive substances and bioadhesives and meniscal repair

The outer and inner meniscus have widely differing repair capability correlating with their relative blood supply [162, 163] (**Figure 1a**). The inner meniscus has the poorest blood supply and consequently the weakest repair response. Many strategies have focussed on the development of measures to improve repair of the inner meniscus and they fall into three broad categories: (i) mesenchymal stem cells administered by direct intra-articular injection; (ii) bioscaffold, hydrogel or bioadhesive cell delivery vehicles for the delivery of chondrocytes, meniscal cells or MSCs into meniscal defects; and (iii) meniscal implants and allografts for total or partial meniscal replacement. These procedures are often undertaken with bioactive substances in the scaffold, hydrogel or bioadhesive delivery system which stimulate repair processes in therapeutic and resident cell populations (**Table 3**). An alternative approach is the co-culture of MSCs with chondrocytes or meniscal cells to pre-condition these or expand cell numbers prior to their incorporation into bioscaffolds, hydrogels or bioadhesives prior to administration to the meniscal defect [159, 164] (**Figure 3a** and **b**). Platelet rich plasma or platelet rich fibrin clots have been used to enhance meniscal repair in bioscaffolds [120, 165–171].

Myoblast loaded PLGA scaffolds have been evaluated for the repair of inner meniscal defects [172]. A derivatised HA, HYADD4® hydrogel cell delivery system has been used for the repair of radial-longitudinal tears in a randomised controlled study [173]. Electrospun type I collagen and gelatin-PLGA bilayered nanofibre reinforced scaffolds seeded with meniscal cells isolated from outer and inner regions have been used in the repair of lesions in the inner meniscus [174, 175] and radio-opaque collagen scaffolds have been used in order to observe the action of therapeutic cells including MSCs on meniscal repair [176]. Meniscal defects wrapped in collagen membranes prior to injection of autologous chondrocytes for repair have been evaluated for the repair of the avascular meniscus [156]. Collagen gel scaffolds containing meniscal, synovial and adipose stem cells have been employed for meniscal repair [177] or in electrospun nanofibrous scaffolds [178]. The use of a type I collagen scaffold and infrapatellar fat pad for meniscal repair has been evaluated in rabbits [179]. PLGA mesh and fibre reinforced collagen-GAG scaffolds seeded with chondrocytes [180] or meniscal cells [168] supplemented with PRP have been evaluated for meniscal repair. Minced juvenile menisci sandwiched with meniscal explants from inner meniscal regions have been evaluated for their reparative potential on tears of the inner meniscal regions [181]. A number of bioactive factors have been evaluated for their reparative properties on meniscal defects. These include multiple injections of leuko-reduced PRP [165], 10% human serum, 5% PRP, 5% autologous plasma [182]. Over expression of TGF-β induced by a rAAV vector, stimulated matrix production and cell proliferation in human meniscal explants consistent with active repair [183]. IGF-I over-expressing meniscal cells induced by transfection of the hIGF-I gene [184] or by liposome Fugene 6 transfer of hIGF-I, stimulated ECM production, proliferation and differentiation of cultured meniscal cells and explants from the inner meniscus [185]. VEGF, BMP-7 and HA stimulated chondrocytes have been implanted into meniscal defects to undertake repair in-vitro [186]. Intra-articular injection of microRNA 210 stimulated mitochondrial activity and angiogenesis promoting repair of avascular meniscal defects by upregulation of anabolic matrix genes by resident meniscal cells, VEGF and FGF-2 production [187]. Fibrin-CTGF administration into avascular defects stimulated repair by the resident meniscal cells [188] as did HA, TGF-β3, platelet concentrates and serum supplemented scaffolds [166, 182, 189]. FGF-2 over-expressing meniscal cells [190, 191] and gelatin-FGF-2 scaffolds [192] also stimulated repair of inner meniscal defects. HA-collagen-PRP composites [47, 193], VEGF [194], TGF-β1 [195] and OP-1 [196] also stimulated meniscal cells and MSCs to undertake repair of inner meniscal defects or punch biopsy wounds in menisci. The bioscaffolds used in meniscal repair or regenerative strategies have been extensively reviewed [197–200].

3.5 Bioadhesives and meniscal repair

First generation fibrin sealant/glue formulations (Tisseel® (Baxter International Inc.), Tissucol® (Baxter Healthcare SA), Beriplast® (CSL Behring GmbH), Hemaseel® (Haemacure Corp)) were originally based on bovine fibrinogen, thrombin and aprotinin isolated from pooled bovine donors. With the discovery of bovine spongiform encephalitis and the technical difficulty of removing prions from bovine protein products, second generation fibrin glues were developed using human proteins and in-house methodologies for the isolation of autologous platelet plasma. Vitagel® (Orthovita Inc.)/Costasis® (Angiotech Pharmaceuticals Inc.) is a fibrin sealant variant containing bovine collagen and thrombin and human plasma. To minimise transmission of viral components, second generation fibrin sealants/glues utilise heat-treated human fibrinogen, autologous platelet plasma and virally incapacitated human thrombin. Autologous fibrin sealants based on platelet rich plasma (PRP), or platelet poor plasma (PPP) with added calcium and thrombin, produce a platelet gel which promotes haemostasis and wound healing aided by the release of platelet growth factors (especially TGF-β1 and TGF-β2) and cytokines. Autologous fibrin sealants suffer inconsistency due to variation in patient plasma protein profiles. Commercial FDA approved second generation fibrin sealants such as Quixil® (OMRIX Biopharmaceuticals SA)/Crosseal™ (OMRIX Biopharmaceuticals) have controlled levels of fibrinogen and thrombin with aprotinin replaced by the anti-fibrinolytic, tranexamic acid. Concerns over the use of tranexamic acid subsequently led to it being dropped from the formulation in the product Evicel® (Ethicon HCP). Formulations of fibrin sealants/glues have been developed as aerosol administered foams and collagen films based on equine collagen and combinations of animal (Tachocomb® (Baxter Healthcare Corp)) and human fibrinogen/thrombin (Tachocomb H®, TachoSil® (Baxter Healthcare Corp)). While fibrin sealants/glues were originally developed to minimise surgical blood loss and to aid in wound repair they have now been applied as autologous cell delivery vehicles for osteochondral repair in autologous chondrocyte implantation (ACI) whereby chondrocyte numbers are expanded in-vitro then loaded into cartilage defects and are contained within this site using a periosteal or collagen membrane sutured over the defect site and sealed along its margins using fibrin sealants/glues. This technique was subsequently modified using the matrix assisted chondrocyte implantation (MACI) procedure where chondrocytes seeded into a matrix material were placed into the chondral defect and sealed in place with fibrin sealant/glue obviating the use of sutures. A modification of this procedure (fibrin ACI) where fibrin sealants were used as scaffolds for cell delivery has also been developed. The fibrin ACI methodology has been applied to the repair of meniscal tears [201–203] using a number of bioactive supplements to improve cell proliferation and matrix synthesis to promote meniscal repair.

An interesting novel bio-glue has been discovered in the Australian frog genus *Notaden bennetti*. During the mating season the female frog expresses an adhesive exudate from the dorsal skin which ensures sexual union with the male for an extended period to ensure effective fertilisation. This exudate has been harvested from frog skin by electro-stimulation and characterised. Examination of the toxicity and biocompatibility of this biological glue [204], its molecular composition and mechanism of action [205] has shown that this protein based adhesive [206] is non-immunogenic, biocompatible, displays elastomeric properties similar to elastin and the strength of its adhesive properties is several fold that of fibrin glue. This frog glue has been used in combination with suturing of infraspinatus tendon to the bone interface in rotator cuff operations and significantly increased the strength of these attachments [207]. The frog glue also outperformed fibrin glue for the re-attachment of the cut surfaces of a longitudinal bucket handle meniscal tear in an in-vitro comparison [208, 209]. Marine sources of biological glues from the New Zealand green lipped mussel and barnacle are known and have appropriate strong adhesive properties for orthopaedic applications, these await commercialisation [210–213].

CS-bone marrow tissue adhesive [214], fibrin stabilised PGA scaffolds [189] have both found application in meniscal repair. New generation bio-glues has been used as cell delivery vehicles and as bioadhesives in meniscal repair [210, 211] and in the re-attachment of horizontal meniscal defects [215]. Mussel based bioadhesives containing antibiotics and fungicides with improved wet strength properties for use in the closure of surgical incisions have even been developed [216, 217].

4. Conclusions

i. Direct MSC-meniscal cell contact and soluble trophic factors both stimulate meniscal repair processes by the resident meniscal cell populations.

ii. The bioscaffolds, hydrogel and bioadhesive cell delivery described in this review provide not only protective matrices for MSC and other administered cells but provide a matrix for attachment of migrating cells at the defect site and physical stabilisation of the defect site to prevent further damage while the repair process ensues. MSCs have impressive therapeutic credentials.

iii. Bioscaffolds and cell delivery systems have undergone significant advances in the last few years facilitating the localisation of MSCs in tissues for reparative purposes, and hold considerable therapeutic promise in the treatment of problematic lesions in the inner meniscus zone.

iv. Many biomaterials have been examined in the quest for potential meniscal implants but none have displayed as efficient properties as the native menisci of the human knee.

v. Clinical trials of partial/total replacement menisci are enrolled and their results are eagerly awaited. Despite promising results, scaffold and implant properties still need optimisation.

vi. Advanced degeneration of menisci and mechanical damage result in a significant loss of meniscal tissue and there is a clear need for a replacement material either for a portion of the meniscus or the meniscus in entirety.

vii. Significant in-roads have been made in the development of new biopolymers for use in 3D printing and slow release biofactors which direct meniscal regeneration.

viii. Developments in bioadhesive design offers improved adhesive properties for surgical applications. These can also be used as cell delivery vehicles to promote meniscal regeneration.

Acknowledgements

NHMRC Project Grant 1004032 funded this study.

Author details

James Melrose[1,2,3,4]*

1 Raymond Purves Bone and Joint Research Laboratory, Kolling Institute, Northern Sydney Local Health District, St. Leonards, NSW, Australia

2 Sydney Medical School, Northern, The University of Sydney, Australia

3 Faculty of Medicine and Health, University of Sydney, Royal North Shore Hospital, St. Leonards, NSW, Australia

4 Graduate School of Biomedical Engineering, University of New South Wales, Sydney, NSW, Australia

*Address all correspondence to: james.melrose@sydney.edu.au

References

[1] Mow V, Ratcliffe A, Chen KY, Kelly MA. Structure and function relationships of the menisci of the knee. In: Mow VC, Arnoczky SP, Jackson DW, editors. Knee Meniscus: Basic and Clinical Foundations. New York: Raven Press; 1992. pp. 37-57

[2] Fithian DC, Kelly MA, Mow VC. Material properties and structure-function relationships in the menisci. Clinical Orthopaedics and Related Research. 1990;**252**:19-31

[3] Ahmed AM, Burke DL. In-vitro measurement of static pressure distribution in synovial joints—part I: Tibial surface of the knee. Journal of Biomechanical Engineering. 1983;**105**:216-225

[4] Walker PS, Erkman MJ. The role of the menisci in force transmission across the knee. Clinical Orthopaedics and Related Research. 1975;**109**:184-192

[5] Tissakht M, Ahmed AM. Tensile stress-strain characteristics of the human meniscal material. Journal of Biomechanics. 1995;**28**:411-422

[6] Storm C, Pastore JJ, MacKintosh FC, Lubensky TC, Janmey PA. Nonlinear elasticity in biological gels. Nature. 2005;**435**:191-194

[7] Makris EA, Hadidi P, Athanasiou KA. The knee meniscus: Structure-function, pathophysiology, current repair techniques, and prospects for regeneration. Biomaterials. 2011;**32**:7411-7431

[8] Lee SJ, Aadalen KJ, Malaviya P, Lorenz EP, Hayden JK, Farr J, Kang RW, Cole BJ. Tibiofemoral contact mechanics after serial medial meniscectomies in the human cadaveric knee. The American Journal of Sports Medicine. 2006;**34**:1334-1344

[9] Cheung HS. Distribution of type I, II, III and V in the pepsin solubilized collagens in bovine menisci. Connective Tissue Research. 1987;**16**:343-356

[10] Gao J. Immunolocalization of types I, II, and X collagen in the tibial insertion sites of the medial meniscus. Knee Surgery, Sports Traumatology, Arthroscopy. 2000;**8**:61-65

[11] Wildey GM, Billetz AC, Matyas JR, Adams ME, McDevitt CA. Absolute concentrations of mRNA for type I and type VI collagen in the canine meniscus in normal and ACL-deficient knee joints obtained by RNase protection assay. Journal of Orthopaedic Research. 2001;**19**:650-658

[12] Eyre DR, Wu JJ. Collagen of fibrocartilage: A distinctive molecular phenotype in bovine meniscus. FEBS Letters. 1983;**158**:265-270

[13] Peterson W, Tillmann B. Collagenous fibril texture of the human knee joint menisci. Anal Embryol. 1998;**197**:317-324

[14] Nakano T, Dodd CM, Scott PG. Glycosaminoglycans and proteoglycans from different zones of the porcine knee meniscus. Journal of Orthopaedic Research. 1997;**15**:213-220

[15] Scott PG, Nakano T, Dodd CM. Isolation and characterization of small proteoglycans from different zones of the porcine knee meniscus. Biochimica et Biophysica Acta. 1997;**1336**:254-262

[16] McAlinden A, Dudhia J, Bolton MC, Lorenzo P, Heinegard D, Bayliss MT. Age-related changes in the synthesis and mRNA expression of decorin and aggrecan in human meniscus and articular cartilage. Osteoarthritis and Cartilage. 2001;**9**:33-41

[17] French MM, Gomes RR Jr, Timpl R, Hook M, Czymmek K, Farach-Carson MC, Carson DD. Chondrogenic activity of the heparan sulfate proteoglycan perlecan maps to the N-terminal domain I. Journal of Bone and Mineral Research. 2002;**17**:48-55

[18] Gomes RR Jr, Farach-Carson MC, Carson DD. Perlecan functions in chondrogenesis: Insights from in vitro and in vivo models. Cells, Tissues, Organs. 2004;**176**:79-86

[19] Yang W, Gomes RR, Brown AJ, Burdett AR, Alicknavitch M, Farach-Carson MC, Carson DD. Chondrogenic differentiation on perlecan domain I, collagen II, and bone morphogenetic protein-2-based matrices. Tissue Engineering. 2006;**12**:2009-2024

[20] Smith SM, Shu C, Melrose J. Comparative immunolocalisation of perlecan with collagen II and aggrecan in human foetal, newborn and adult ovine joint tissues demonstrates perlecan as an early developmental chondrogenic marker. Histochemistry and Cell Biology. 2010;**134**:251-263

[21] Englund M, Guermazi A, Lohmander LS. The meniscus in knee osteoarthritis. Rheumatic Diseases Clinics of North America. 2009;**35**:579-590

[22] Englund M, Guermazi A, Lohmander SL. The role of the meniscus in knee osteoarthritis: A cause or consequence? Radiologic Clinics of North America. 2009;**47**:703-712

[23] Brown S, Matta A, Erwin M, Roberts S, Gruber HE, Hanley EN Jr, Little CB, Melrose J. Cell clusters are indicative of stem cell activity in the degenerate intervertebral disc: Can their properties be manipulated to improve intrinsic repair of the disc? Stem Cells and Development. 2018;**27**:147-165

[24] Jayasuriya CT, Hu N, Li J, Lemme N, Terek R, Ehrlich MG, Chen Q. Molecular characterization of mesenchymal stem cells in human osteoarthritis cartilage reveals contribution to the OA phenotype. Scientific Reports. 2018;**8**:7044

[25] McGonagle D, Baboolal TG, Jones E. Native joint-resident mesenchymal stem cells for cartilage repair in osteoarthritis. Nature Reviews Rheumatology. 2017;**13**:719-730

[26] Tesche F, Miosge N. Perlecan in late stages of osteoarthritis of the human knee joint. Osteoarthritis and Cartilage. 2004;**12**:852-862

[27] Tesche F, Miosge N. New aspects of the pathogenesis of osteoarthritis: The role of fibroblast-like chondrocytes in late stages of the disease. Histology and Histopathology. 2005;**20**:329-337

[28] Turner S, Balain B, Caterson B, Morgan C, Roberts S. Viability, growth kinetics and stem cell markers of single and clustered cells in human intervertebral discs: Implications for regenerative therapies. European Spine Journal. 2014;**23**:2462-2472

[29] Franceschetti T, De Bari C. The potential role of adult stem cells in the management of the rheumatic diseases. Therapeutic Advances in Musculoskeletal Disease. 2017;**9**:165-179

[30] Shu C, Fuller E, Melrose J. Co-culture of mesenchymal stromal stem and meniscal cells upregulates type I and type II collagen and aggrecan production conducive to meniscal repair. Current Topics in Biotechnology. 2018;**9**:11-20

[31] Caplan AI. Mesenchymal stem cells. Journal of Orthopaedic Research. 1991;**9**:641-650

[32] Caplan AI. Review: Mesenchymal stem cells: Cell-based reconstructive therapy in orthopedics. Tissue Engineering. 2005;**11**:1198-1211

[33] Caplan AI. Why are MSCs therapeutic? New data: New insight. Journal of Pathology. 2009;**217**:318-324

[34] Caplan AI. MSCs: The sentinel and safe-guards of injury. Journal of Cellular Physiology. 2016;**231**:1413-1416

[35] Baglio SR, Pegtel DM, Baldini N. Mesenchymal stem cell secreted vesicles provide novel opportunities in (stem) cell-free therapy. Frontiers in Physiology. 2012;**3**:359

[36] Bobis-Wozowicz S, Kmiotek K, Sekula M, Kedracka-Krok S, Kamycka E, Adamiak M, Jankowska U, Madetko-Talowska A, Sarna M, Bik-Multanowski M, Kolcz J, Boruczkowski D, Madeja Z, Dawn B, Zuba-Surma EK. Human induced pluripotent stem cell-derived microvesicles transmit RNAs and proteins to recipient mature heart cells modulating cell fate and behavior. Stem Cells. 2015;**33**:2748-2761

[37] Boomsma RA, Geenen DL. Evidence for transfer of membranes from mesenchymal stem cells to HL-1 cardiac cells. Stem Cells International. 2014;**2014**:653734

[38] Choi HY, Moon SJ, Ratliff BB, Ahn SH, Jung A, Lee M, Lee S, Lim BJ, Kim BS, Plotkin MD, Ha SK, Park HC. Microparticles from kidney-derived mesenchymal stem cells act as carriers of proangiogenic signals and contribute to recovery from acute kidney injury. PLoS One. 2014;**9**:e87853

[39] da Silva Meirelles L, Caplan AI, Nardi NB. In search of the in vivo identity of mesenchymal stem cells. Stem Cells. 2008;**26**:2287-2299

[40] Devine SM, Peter S, Martin BJ, Barry F, McIntosh KR. Mesenchymal stem cells: Stealth and suppression. Cancer Journal. 2001;**7**(Suppl 2):S76-S82

[41] Gao Y, Lu Z, Chen C, Cui X, Liu Y, Zheng T, Jiang X, Zeng C, Quan D, Wang Q. Mesenchymal stem cells and endothelial progenitor cells accelerate intra-aneurysmal tissue organization after treatment with SDF-1alpha-coated coils. Neurological Research. 2016;**38**:1-9

[42] Melrose J. Strategies in regenerative medicine for intervertebral disc repair using mesenchymal stem cells and bioscaffolds. Regenerative Medicine. 2016;**11**:705-724

[43] Xie X, Zhu J, Hu X, Dai L, Fu X, Zhang J, Duan X, Ao Y. A co-culture system of rat synovial stem cells and meniscus cells promotes cell proliferation and differentiation as compared to mono-culture. Scientific Reports. 2018;**8**:7693

[44] Angele P, Kujat R, Koch M, Zellner J. Role of mesenchymal stem cells in meniscal repair. Journal of Experimental Orthopaedics. 2014;**1**:12

[45] Yu H, Adesida AB, Jomha NM. Meniscus repair using mesenchymal stem cells—A comprehensive review. Stem Cell Research & Therapy. 2015;**6**:86

[46] Zellner J, Hierl K, Mueller M, Pfeifer C, Berner A, Dienstknecht T, Krutsch W, Geis S, Gehmert S, Kujat R, Dendorfer S, Prantl L, Nerlich M, Angele P. Stem cell-based tissue-engineering for treatment of meniscal tears in the avascular zone. Journal of Biomedical Materials Research. Part B, Applied Biomaterials. 2013;**101**:1133-1142

[47] Zellner J, Mueller M, Berner A, Dienstknecht T, Kujat R, Nerlich M, Hennemann B, Koller M, Prantl L, Angele M, Angele P. Role of mesenchymal stem cells in tissue engineering of meniscus. Journal of Biomedical Materials Research. Part A. 2010;**94**:1150-1161

[48] Zellner J, Pattappa G, Koch M, Lang S, Weber J, Pfeifer CG, Mueller MB, Kujat R, Nerlich M, Angele P.

Autologous mesenchymal stem cells or meniscal cells: What is the best cell source for regenerative meniscus treatment in an early osteoarthritis situation? Stem Cell Research & Therapy. 2017;**8**:225

[49] Appleyard RC, Burkhardt D, Ghosh P, Read R, Cake M, Swain MV, Murrell GA. Topographical analysis of the structural, biochemical and dynamic biomechanical properties of cartilage in an ovine model of osteoarthritis. Osteoarthritis and Cartilage. 2003;**11**:65-77

[50] Appleyard RC, Ghosh P, Swain MV. Biomechanical, histological and immunohistological studies of patellar cartilage in an ovine model of osteoarthritis induced by lateral meniscectomy. Osteoarthritis and Cartilage. 1999;**7**:281-294

[51] Armstrong S, Read R, Ghosh P. The effects of intraarticular hyaluronan on cartilage and subchondral bone changes in an ovine model of early osteoarthritis. The Journal of Rheumatology. 1994;**21**:680-688

[52] Bulgheroni P, Bulgheroni E, Regazzola G, Mazzola C. Polyurethane scaffold for the treatment of partial meniscal tears. Clinical results with a minimum two-year follow-up. Joints. 2013;**1**:161-166

[53] Burkhardt D, Hwa SY, Ghosh P. A novel microassay for the quantitation of the sulfated glycosaminoglycan content of histological sections: Its application to determine the effects of Diacerhein on cartilage in an ovine model of osteoarthritis. Osteoarthritis and Cartilage. 2001;**9**:238-247

[54] Cake M, Read R, Edwards S, Smith MM, Burkhardt D, Little C, Ghosh P. Changes in gait after bilateral meniscectomy in sheep: Effect of two hyaluronan preparations. Journal of Orthopaedic Science. 2008;**13**:514-523

[55] Cake MA, Read RA, Appleyard RC, Hwa SY, Ghosh P. The nitric oxide donor glyceryl trinitrate increases subchondral bone sclerosis and cartilage degeneration following ovine meniscectomy. Osteoarthritis and Cartilage. 2004;**12**:974-981

[56] Cake MA, Read RA, Corfield G, Daniel A, Burkhardt D, Smith MM, Little CB. Comparison of gait and pathology outcomes of three meniscal procedures for induction of knee osteoarthritis in sheep. Osteoarthritis and Cartilage. 2013;**21**:226-236

[57] Cake MA, Read RA, Guillou B, Ghosh P. Modification of articular cartilage and subchondral bone pathology in an ovine meniscectomy model of osteoarthritis by avocado and soya unsaponifiables (ASU). Osteoarthritis and Cartilage. 2000;**8**:404-411

[58] Cake MA, Smith MM, Young AA, Smith SM, Ghosh P, Read RA. Synovial pathology in an ovine model of osteoarthritis: Effect of intraarticular hyaluronan (Hyalgan). Clinical and Experimental Rheumatology. 2008;**26**:561-567

[59] Chatain F, Robinson AH, Adeleine P, Chambat P, Neyret P. The natural history of the knee following arthroscopic medial meniscectomy. Knee Surgery, Sports Traumatology, Arthroscopy. 2001;**9**:15-18

[60] Englund M. The role of the meniscus in osteoarthritis genesis. Rheumatic Diseases Clinics of North America. 2008;**34**:573-579

[61] Englund M. The role of the meniscus in osteoarthritis genesis. The Medical Clinics of North America. 2009;**93**:37-43

[62] Ghosh P, Holbert C, Read R, Armstrong S. Hyaluronic acid (hyaluronan) in experimental osteoarthritis. The Journal of

Rheumatology. Supplement. 1995;**43**:155-157

[63] Ghosh P, Read R, Numata Y, Smith S, Armstrong S, Wilson D. The effects of intraarticular administration of hyaluronan in a model of early osteoarthritis in sheep. II. Cartilage composition and proteoglycan metabolism. Seminars in Arthritis and Rheumatism. 1993;**22**:31-42

[64] Hwa SY, Burkhardt D, Little C, Ghosh P. The effects of orally administered diacerein on cartilage and subchondral bone in an ovine model of osteoarthritis. The Journal of Rheumatology. 2001;**28**:825-834

[65] Jarraya M, Roemer FW, Englund M, Crema MD, Gale HI, Hayashi D, Katz JN, Guermazi A. Meniscus morphology: Does tear type matter? A narrative review with focus on relevance for osteoarthritis research. Seminars in Arthritis and Rheumatism. 2017;**46**:552-561

[66] Little C, Smith S, Ghosh P, Bellenger C. Histomorphological and immunohistochemical evaluation of joint changes in a model of osteoarthritis induced by lateral meniscectomy in sheep. The Journal of Rheumatology. 1997;**24**:2199-2209

[67] McDaniel D, Tilton E, Dominick K, Flory K, Ernest T, Johnson JC, Main DC, Kondrashov P. Histological characteristics of knee menisci in patients with osteoarthritis. Clinical Anatomy. 2017;**30**:805-810

[68] Oakley SP, Lassere MN, Portek I, Szomor Z, Ghosh P, Kirkham BW, Murrell GA, Wulf S, Appleyard RC. Biomechanical, histologic and macroscopic assessment of articular cartilage in a sheep model of osteoarthritis. Osteoarthritis and Cartilage. 2004;**12**:667-679

[69] Oakley SP, Portek I, Szomor Z, Appleyard RC, Ghosh P, Kirkham BW, Murrell GA, Lassere MN. Arthroscopy—A potential "gold standard" for the diagnosis of the chondropathy of early osteoarthritis. Osteoarthritis and Cartilage. 2005;**13**:368-378

[70] Shakespeare DT, Rigby HS. The bucket-handle tear of the meniscus. A clinical and arthrographic study. Journal of Bone and Joint Surgery. 1983;**65**:383-387

[71] Smith MM, Cake MA, Ghosh P, Schiavinato A, Read RA, Little CB. Significant synovial pathology in a meniscectomy model of osteoarthritis: Modification by intra-articular hyaluronan therapy. Rheumatology (Oxford, England). 2008;**47**:1172-1178

[72] Tasker T, Waugh W. Articular changes associated with internal derangement of the knee. Journal of Bone and Joint Surgery. British Volume (London). 1982;**64**:486-488

[73] Young AA, Smith MM, Smith SM, Cake MA, Ghosh P, Read RA, Melrose J, Sonnabend DH, Roughley PJ, Little CB. Regional assessment of articular cartilage gene expression and small proteoglycan metabolism in an animal model of osteoarthritis. Arthritis Research & Therapy. 2005;7:R852-R861

[74] Ghosh P, Read R, Armstrong S, Wilson D, Marshall R, McNair P. The effects of intraarticular administration of hyaluronan in a model of early osteoarthritis in sheep. I. Gait analysis and radiological and morphological studies. Seminars in Arthritis and Rheumatism. 1993;**22**:18-30

[75] Seil R, Becker R. Time for a paradigm change in meniscal repair: Save the meniscus! Knee Surgery, Sports Traumatology, Arthroscopy. 2016;**24**:1421-1423

[76] Beaufils P, Becker R, Kopf S, Englund M, Verdonk R, Ollivier M, Seil R.

Surgical management of degenerative meniscus lesions: The 2016 ESSKA meniscus consensus. Joints. 2017;**5**:59-69

[77] Little CB, Ghosh P, Bellenger CR. Topographic variation in biglycan and decorin synthesis by articular cartilage in the early stages of osteoarthritis: An experimental study in sheep. Journal of Orthopaedic Research. 1996;**14**:433-444

[78] Melrose J, Smith S, Cake M, Read R, Whitelock J. Comparative spatial and temporal localisation of perlecan, aggrecan and type I, II and IV collagen in the ovine meniscus: An ageing study. Histochemistry and Cell Biolog. 2005;**124**:225-235

[79] Young AA, McLennan S, Smith MM, Smith SM, Cake MA, Read RA, Melrose J, Sonnabend DH, Flannery CR, Little CB. Proteoglycan 4 downregulation in a sheep meniscectomy model of early osteoarthritis. Arthritis Research & Therapy. 2006;**8**:R41

[80] Melrose J, Fuller ES, Roughley PJ, Smith MM, Kerr B, Hughes CE, Caterson B, Little CB. Fragmentation of decorin, biglycan, lumican and keratocan is elevated in degenerate human meniscus, knee and hip articular cartilages compared with age-matched macroscopically normal and control tissues. Arthritis Research & Therapy. 2008;**10**:R79

[81] Fuller E, Little CB, Melrose J. Interleukin-1alpha induces focal degradation of biglycan and tissue degeneration in an in-vitro ovine meniscal model. Experimental and Molecular Pathology. 2016;**101**:214-220

[82] Fuller ES, Smith MM, Little CB, Melrose J. Zonal differences in meniscus matrix turnover and cytokine response. Osteoarthritis and Cartilage. 2012;**20**:49-59

[83] Melrose J, Fuller EM, Little CB. The biology of meniscal pathology in osteoarthritis and its contribution to joint disease: Beyond simple mechanics. Connective Tissue Research. 2016, 2017;**58**(3-4):282-294

[84] Zaffagnini S, Grassi A, Marcheggiani Muccioli GM, Holsten D, Bulgheroni P, Monllau JC, Berbig R, Lagae K, Crespo R, Marcacci M. Two-year clinical results of lateral collagen meniscus implant: A multicenter study. Arthroscopy. 2015;**31**:1269-1278

[85] Bouyarmane H, Beaufils P, Pujol N, Bellemans J, Roberts S, Spalding T, Zaffagnini S, Marcacci M, Verdonk P, Womack M, Verdonk R. Polyurethane scaffold in lateral meniscus segmental defects: Clinical outcomes at 24 months follow-up. Orthopaedics & Traumatology, Surgery & Research. 2014;**100**:153-157

[86] Vrancken AC, Buma P, van Tienen TG. Synthetic meniscus replacement: A review. International Orthopaedics. 2013;**37**:291-299

[87] Hansen R, Choi G, Bryk E, Vigorita V. The human knee meniscus: A review with special focus on the collagen meniscal implant. Journal of Long-Term Effects of Medical Implants. 2011;**21**:321-337

[88] Baynat C, Andro C, Vincent JP, Schiele P, Buisson P, Dubrana F, Gunepin FX. Actifit synthetic meniscal substitute: Experience with 18 patients in Brest, France. Orthopaedics & Traumatology: Surgery & Research. 2014;**100**:S385-S389

[89] Dhollander A, Verdonk P, Verdonk R. Treatment of painful, irreparable partial meniscal defects with a polyurethane scaffold: Midterm clinical outcomes and survival analysis. The American Journal of Sports Medicine. 2016;**44**:2615-2621

[90] Schuttler KF, Haberhauer F, Gesslein M, Heyse TJ, Figiel J, Lorbach O, Efe T, Roessler PP. Midterm follow-up after implantation of a polyurethane

meniscal scaffold for segmental medial meniscus loss: Maintenance of good clinical and MRI outcome. Knee Surgery, Sports Traumatology, Arthroscopy. 2016;**24**:1478-1484

[91] De Coninck T, Elsner JJ, Linder-Ganz E, Cromheecke M, Shemesh M, Huysse W, Verdonk R, Verstraete K, Verdonk P. In-vivo evaluation of the kinematic behavior of an artificial medial meniscus implant: A pilot study using open-MRI. Clinical Biomechanics (Bristol, Avon). 2014;**29**:898-905

[92] Elsner JJ, Portnoy S, Zur G, Guilak F, Shterling A, Linder-Ganz E. Design of a free-floating polycarbonate-urethane meniscal implant using finite element modeling and experimental validation. Journal of Biomechanical Engineering. 2010;**132**:095001

[93] Zur G, Linder-Ganz E, Elsner JJ, Shani J, Brenner O, Agar G, Hershman EB, Arnoczky SP, Guilak F, Shterling A. Chondroprotective effects of a polycarbonate-urethane meniscal implant: Histopathological results in a sheep model. Knee Surgery, Sports Traumatology, Arthroscopy. 2011;**19**:255-263

[94] Kaleka CC, Debieux P, da Costa Astur D, Arliani GG, Cohen M. Updates in biological therapies for knee injuries: Menisci. Current Reviews in Musculoskeletal Medicine. 2014;7:247-255

[95] Hayes JC, Curley C, Tierney P, Kennedy JE. Biomechanical analysis of a salt-modified polyvinyl alcohol hydrogel for knee meniscus applications, including comparison with human donor samples. Journal of the Mechanical Behavior of Biomedical Materials. 2016;**56**:156-164

[96] Yoo JJ, Bichara DA, Zhao X, Randolph MA, Gill TJ. Implant-assisted meniscal repair in vivo using a chondrocyte-seeded flexible PLGA scaffold. Journal of Biomedical Materials Research. Part A. 2011;**99**:102-108

[97] Lu HD, Cai DZ, Wu G, Wang K, Shi DH. Whole meniscus regeneration using polymer scaffolds loaded with fibrochondrocytes. Chinese Journal of Traumatology. 2011;**14**:195-204

[98] Tienen TG, Heijkants RG, de Groot JH, Pennings AJ, Schouten AJ, Veth RP, Buma P. Replacement of the knee meniscus by a porous polymer implant: A study in dogs. The American Journal of Sports Medicine. 2006;**34**:64-71

[99] Buma P, van Tienen T, Veth R. The collagen meniscus implant. Expert Review of Medical Devices. 2007;**4**:507-516

[100] Frank RM, Cole BJ. Meniscus transplantation. Current Reviews in Musculoskeletal Medicine. 2015;**8**:443-450

[101] Lin DD, Picardo NE, Adesida A, Khan WS. Clinical studies using biological and synthetic materials for meniscus replacement. Current Stem Cell Research & Therapy. 2016;**12**:348-353

[102] Bakarich SE, Gorkin R 3rd, In Het Panhuis M, Spinks GM. Three-dimensional printing fiber reinforced hydrogel composites. ACS Applied Materials & Interfaces. 2014;**6**:15998-16006

[103] Szoika A, Lalh K, Andrews SHJ, Jomha NM, Osswald M, Adesida AB. Biomimetic 3D printed scaffolds for meniscus tissue engineering. Bioprinting. 2017;**8**:1-7

[104] Yang F, Tadapelli V, Wiley BJ. 3D printing of a double network hydrogel with a compression strength and elastic Modulus greater than those of cartilage ACS. Biomaterials. 2017;**3**:863-869

[105] Zhang ZZ, Wang SJ, Zhang JY, Jiang WB, Huang AB, Qi YS, Ding JX,

Chen XS, Jiang D, Yu JK. 3D-printed poly(epsilon-caprolactone) scaffold augmented with mesenchymal stem cells for total meniscal substitution: A 12- and 24-week animal study in a rabbit model. The American Journal of Sports Medicine. 2017;**45**:1497-1511

[106] Lee CH, Rodeo SA, Fortier LA, Lu C, Erisken C, Mao JJ. Protein-releasing polymeric scaffolds induce fibrochondrocytic differentiation of endogenous cells for knee meniscus regeneration in sheep. Science Translational Medicine. 2014;**6**:266ra171

[107] Spees JL, Lee RH, Gregory CA. Mechanisms of mesenchymal stem/stromal cell function. Stem Cell Research & Therapy. 2016;7:125

[108] Shi X, Liu J, Yang T, Zhang Y, Li T, Chen J. TLR2/NFkappaB signalling regulates endogenous IL-6 release from marrow-derived mesenchymal stromal cells to suppress the apoptosis of PC12 cells injured by oxygen and glucose deprivation. Molecular Medicine Reports. 2016;**13**:5358-5364

[109] Song YS, Joo HW, Park IH, Shen GY, Lee Y, Shin JH, Kim H, Kim KS. Bone marrow mesenchymal stem cell-derived vascular endothelial growth factor attenuates cardiac apoptosis via regulation of cardiac miRNA-23a and miRNA-92a in a rat model of myocardial infarction. PLoS One. 2017;**12**:e0179972

[110] Bifari F, Lisi V, Mimiola E, Pasini A, Krampera M. Immune modulation by mesenchymal stem cells. Transfusion Medicine and Hemotherapy. 2008;**35**:194-204

[111] Bruno S, Deregibus MC, Camussi G. The secretome of mesenchymal stromal cells: Role of extracellular vesicles in immunomodulation. Immunology Letters. 2015;**168**:154-158

[112] Caplan AI, Sorrell JM. The MSC curtain that stops the immune system. Immunology Letters. 2015;**168**:136-139

[113] Fibbe WE, Nauta AJ, Roelofs H. Modulation of immune responses by mesenchymal stem cells. Annals of the New York Academy of Sciences. 2007;**1106**:272-278

[114] Rasmusson I. Immune modulation by mesenchymal stem cells. Experimental Cell Research. 2006;**312**:2169-2179

[115] Caplan AI. Mesenchymal stem cells: Time to change the name! Stem Cells Translational Medicine. 2017;**6**:1445-1451

[116] Trounson A, McDonald C. Stem cell therapies in clinical trials: Progress and challenges. Cell Stem Cell. 2015;**17**:11-22

[117] Barry F, Murphy JM, O-Brien T, Mahon B. Mesenchymal stem cell transplantation for tissue repair. Seminars in Plastic Surgery. 2005;**19**:229-239

[118] Ansari S, Chen C, Xu X, Annabi N, Zadeh HH, Wu BM, Khademhosseini A, Shi S, Moshaverinia A. Muscle tissue engineering using gingival mesenchymal stem cells encapsulated in alginate hydrogels containing multiple growth factors. Annals of Biomedical Engineering. 2016;**44**:1908-1920

[119] Hellstrom M, Moreno-Moya JM, Bandstein S, Bom E, Akouri RR, Miyazaki K, Maruyama T, Brannstrom M. Bioengineered uterine tissue supports pregnancy in a rat model. Fertility and Sterility. 2016;**106**:487-496

[120] Hutchinson ID, Rodeo SA, Perrone GS, Murray MM. Can platelet-rich plasma enhance anterior cruciate ligament and meniscal repair? The Journal of Knee Surgery. 2015;**28**:19-28

[121] Murphy M, Barry F. Cellular chondroplasty: A new technology for joint regeneration. The Journal of Knee Surgery. 2015;**28**:45-50

[122] Ozpur MA, Guneren E, Canter HI, Karaaltin MV, Ovali E, Yogun FN,

Baygol EG, Kaplan S. Generation of skin tissue using adipose tissue-derived stem cells. Plastic and Reconstructive Surgery. 2016;**137**:134-143

[123] Pantcheva P, Reyes S, Hoover J, Kaelber S, Borlongan CV. Treating non-motor symptoms of Parkinson's disease with transplantation of stem cells. Expert Review of Neurotherapeutics. 2015;**15**:1231-1240

[124] Saini JS, Temple S, Stern JH. Human retinal pigment epithelium stem cell (RPESC). Advances in Experimental Medicine and Biology. 2016;**854**:557-562

[125] Tilokee EL, Latham N, Jackson R, Mayfield AE, Ye B, Mount S, Lam BK, Suuronen EJ, Ruel M, Stewart DJ, Davis DR. Paracrine engineering of human explant-derived cardiac stem cells to over-express stromal-cell derived factor 1alpha enhances myocardial repair. Stem Cells. 2016;**34**:1826-1835

[126] Abumaree M, Al Jumah M, Pace RA, Kalionis B. Immunosuppressive properties of mesenchymal stem cells. Stem Cell Reviews. 2012;**8**:375-392

[127] Dimarino AM, Caplan AI, Bonfield TL. Mesenchymal stem cells in tissue repair. Frontiers in Immunology. 2013;**4**:201

[128] Parekkadan B, Milwid JM. Mesenchymal stem cells as therapeutics. Annual Review of Biomedical Engineering. 2010;**12**:87-117

[129] Prockop DJ, Oh JY. Mesenchymal stem/stromal cells (MSCs): Role as guardians of inflammation. Molecular Therapy. 2012;**20**:14-20

[130] Vizoso FJ, Eiro N, Cid S, Schneider J, Perez-Fernandez R. Mesenchymal stem cell secretome: Toward cell-free therapeutic strategies in regenerative medicine. International Journal of Molecular Sciences. 2017;**18**. pii: E1852

[131] Ansboro S, Greiser U, Barry F, Murphy M. Strategies for improved targeting of therapeutic cells: Implications for tissue repair. European Cells & Materials. 2012;**23**:310-318 discussion 318-319

[132] Caplan AI, Dennis JE. Mesenchymal stem cells as trophic mediators. Journal of Cellular Biochemistry. 2006;**98**:1076-1084

[133] Caplan AI. Mesenchymal stem cells: The past, the present, the future. Cartilage. 2010;**1**:6-9

[134] Caplan AI. Adult mesenchymal stem cells: When, where, and how. Stem Cells International. 2015;**2015**:628767

[135] Barry F, Murphy M. Mesenchymal stem cells in joint disease and repair. Nature Reviews Rheumatology. 2013;**9**:584-594

[136] Guescini M, Guidolin D, Vallorani L, Casadei L, Gioacchini AM, Tibollo P, Battistelli M, Falcieri E, Battistin L, Agnati LF, Stocchi V. C2C12 myoblasts release micro-vesicles containing mtDNA and proteins involved in signal transduction. Experimental Cell Research. 2010;**316**:1977-1984

[137] Yang J, Liu XX, Fan H, Tang Q, Shou ZX, Zuo DM, Zou Z, Xu M, Chen QY, Peng Y, Deng SJ, Liu YJ. Extracellular vesicles derived from bone marrow mesenchymal stem cells protect against experimental colitis via attenuating colon inflammation, oxidative stress and apoptosis. PLoS One. 2015;**10**:e0140551

[138] Ong E, Chimutengwende-Gordon M, Khan W. Stem cell therapy for knee ligament, articular cartilage and meniscal injuries. Current Stem Cell Research & Therapy. 2013;**8**:422-428

[139] Pereira H, Frias AM, Oliveira JM, Espregueira-Mendes J, Reis RL. Tissue engineering and regenerative medicine

strategies in meniscus lesions. Arthroscopy. 2011;**27**:1706-1719

[140] Scordino LE, Deberardino TM. Biologic enhancement of meniscus repair. Clinics in Sports Medicine. 2012;**31**:91-100

[141] Vangsness CT Jr, Farr J 2nd, Boyd J, Dellaero DT, Mills CR, LeRoux-Williams M. Adult human mesenchymal stem cells delivered via intra-articular injection to the knee following partial medial meniscectomy: A randomized, double-blind, controlled study. The Journal of Bone and Joint Surgery. American Volume. 2014;**96**:90-98

[142] Horie M, Driscoll MD, Sampson HW, Sekiya I, Caroom CT, Prockop DJ, Thomas DB. Implantation of allogenic synovial stem cells promotes meniscal regeneration in a rabbit meniscal defect model. The Journal of Bone and Joint Surgery. American Volume. 2012;**94**:701-712

[143] Horie M, Sekiya I, Muneta T, Ichinose S, Matsumoto K, Saito H, Murakami T, Kobayashi E. Intra-articular injected synovial stem cells differentiate into meniscal cells directly and promote meniscal regeneration without mobilization to distant organs in rat massive meniscal defect. Stem Cells. 2009;**27**:878-887

[144] Moriguchi Y, Tateishi K, Ando W, Shimomura K, Yonetani Y, Tanaka Y, Kita K, Hart DA, Gobbi A, Shino K, Yoshikawa H, Nakamura N. Repair of meniscal lesions using a scaffold-free tissue-engineered construct derived from allogenic synovial MSCs in a miniature swine model. Biomaterials. 2013;**34**:2185-2193

[145] Nakagawa Y, Muneta T, Kondo S, Mizuno M, Takakuda K, Ichinose S, Tabuchi T, Koga H, Tsuji K, Sekiya I. Synovial mesenchymal stem cells promote healing after meniscal repair in microminipigs. Osteoarthritis and Cartilage. 2015;**23**:1007-1017

[146] Qi Y, Yang Z, Ding Q, Zhao T, Huang Z, Feng G. Targeted transplantation of iron oxide-labeled, adipose-derived mesenchymal stem cells in promoting meniscus regeneration following a rabbit massive meniscal defect. Experimental and Therapeutic Medicine. 2016;**11**:458-466

[147] Toratani T, Nakase J, Numata H, Oshima T, Takata Y, Nakayama K, Tsuchiya H. Scaffold-free tissue-engineered allogenic adipose-derived stem cells promote meniscus healing. Arthroscopy. 2017;**33**:346-354

[148] Ding Z, Huang H. Mesenchymal stem cells in rabbit meniscus and bone marrow exhibit a similar feature but a heterogeneous multi-differentiation potential: Superiority of meniscus as a cell source for meniscus repair. BMC Musculoskeletal Disorders. 2015;**16**:65

[149] Ferris D, Frisbie D, Kisiday J, McIlwraith CW. In vivo healing of meniscal lacerations using bone marrow-derived mesenchymal stem cells and fibrin glue. Stem Cells International. 2012;**2012**:691605

[150] Yoo JU, Barthel TS, Nishimura K, Solchaga L, Caplan AI, Goldberg VM, Johnstone B. The chondrogenic potential of human bone-marrow-derived mesenchymal progenitor cells. The Journal of Bone and Joint Surgery. American Volume. 1998;**80**:1745-1757

[151] Osawa A, Harner CD, Gharaibeh B, Matsumoto T, Mifune Y, Kopf S, Ingham SJ, Schreiber V, Usas A, Huard J. The use of blood vessel-derived stem cells for meniscal regeneration and repair. Medicine and Science in Sports and Exercise. 2013;**45**:813-823

[152] Chew E, Prakash R, Khan W. Mesenchymal stem cells in human meniscal regeneration: A systematic review. Annals of Medicine and Surgery. 2017;**24**:3-7

[153] Pak J, Lee JH, Park KS, Jeon JH, Lee SH. Potential use of mesenchymal stem

cells in human meniscal repair: Current insights. Open Access Journal of Sports Medicine. 2017;**8**:33-38

[154] Niu W, Guo W, Han S, Zhu Y, Liu S, Guo Q. Cell-based strategies for meniscus tissue engineering. Stem Cells International. 2016;**2016**:4717184

[155] Huang H, Wang S, Gui J, Shen H. A study to identify and characterize the stem/progenitor cell in rabbit meniscus. Cytotechnology. 2016;**68**:2083-2103

[156] Julke H, Mainil-Varlet P, Jakob RP, Brehm W, Schafer B, Nesic D. The role of cells in meniscal guided tissue regeneration: A proof of concept study in a goat model. Cartilage. 2015;**6**:20-29

[157] Whitehouse MR, Howells NR, Parry MC, Austin E, Kafienah W, Brady K, Goodship AE, Eldridge JD, Blom AW, Hollander AP. Repair of torn avascular meniscal cartilage using undifferentiated autologous mesenchymal stem cells: From in vitro optimization to a first-in-human study. Stem Cells Translational Medicine. 2017;**6**:1237-1248

[158] Yuan X, Wei Y, Villasante A, Ng JJD, Arkonac DE, Chao PG, Vunjak-Novakovic G. Stem cell delivery in tissue-specific hydrogel enabled meniscal repair in an orthotopic rat model. Biomaterials. 2017;**132**:59-71

[159] McCorry MC, Puetzer JL, Bonassar LJ. Characterization of mesenchymal stem cells and fibrochondrocytes in three-dimensional co-culture: Analysis of cell shape, matrix production, and mechanical performance. Stem Cell Research & Therapy. 2016;**7**:39

[160] Kremer A, Ribitsch I, Reboredo J, Durr J, Egerbacher M, Jenner F, Walles H. Three-dimensional coculture of meniscal cells and mesenchymal stem cells in collagen type I hydrogel on a small intestinal matrix—A pilot study toward equine meniscus tissue engineering. Tissue Engineering. Part A. 2017;**23**:390-402

[161] Farrugia BL, Lord MS, Whitelock JM, Melrose J. Harnessing chondroitin sulphate in composite scaffolds to direct progenitor and stem cell function for tissue repair. Biomaterials Science. 2018;**6**:947-957

[162] Arnoczky SP, Warren RF. Microvasculature of the human meniscus. The American Journal of Sports Medicine. 1982;**10**:90-95

[163] Kobayashi K, Fujimoto E, Deie M, Sumen Y, Ikuta Y, Ochi M. Regional differences in the healing potential of the meniscus-an organ culture model to eliminate the influence of microvasculature and the synovium. The Knee. 2004;**11**:271-278

[164] Cui X, Hasegawa A, Lotz M, D'Lima D. Structured three-dimensional co-culture of mesenchymal stem cells with meniscus cells promotes meniscal phenotype without hypertrophy. Biotechnology and Bioengineering. 2012;**109**:2369-2380

[165] Cook JL, Smith PA, Bozynski CC, Kuroki K, Cook CR, Stoker AM, Pfeiffer FM. Multiple injections of leukoreduced platelet rich plasma reduce pain and functional impairment in a canine model of ACL and meniscal deficiency. Journal of Orthopaedic Research. 2016;**34**:607-615

[166] Freymann U, Metzlaff S, Kruger JP, Hirsh G, Endres M, Petersen W, Kaps C. Effect of human serum and 2 different types of platelet concentrates on human meniscus cell migration, proliferation, and matrix formation. Arthroscopy. 2016;**32**:1106-1116

[167] Griffin JW, Hadeed MM, Werner BC, Diduch DR, Carson EW, Miller MD. Platelet-rich plasma in meniscal repair: Does augmentation improve surgical outcomes? Clinical Orthopaedics and Related Research. 2015;**473**:1665-1672

[168] Howard D, Shepherd JH, Kew SJ, Hernandez P, Ghose S, Wardale JA,

Rushton N. Release of growth factors from a reinforced collagen GAG matrix supplemented with platelet rich plasma: Influence on cultured human meniscal cells. Journal of Orthopaedic Research. 2014;**32**:273-278

[169] Kaminski R, Kulinski K, Kozar-Kaminska K, Wielgus M, Langner M, Wasko MK, Kowalczewski J, Pomianowski S. A prospective, randomized, double-blind, parallel-group, placebo-controlled study evaluating meniscal healing, clinical outcomes, and safety in patients undergoing meniscal repair of unstable, complete vertical meniscal tears (bucket handle) augmented with platelet-rich plasma. BioMed Research International. 2018;**2018**:9315815

[170] Kwak HS, Nam J, Lee JH, Kim HJ, Yoo JJ. Meniscal repair in vivo using human chondrocyte-seeded PLGA mesh scaffold pretreated with platelet-rich plasma. Journal of Tissue Engineering and Regenerative Medicine. 2017;**11**:471-480

[171] Pujol N, Salle De Chou E, Boisrenoult P, Beaufils P. Platelet-rich plasma for open meniscal repair in young patients: Any benefit? Knee Surgery, Sports Traumatology, Arthroscopy. 2015;**23**:51-58

[172] Gu Y, Zhu W, Hao Y, Lu L, Chen Y, Wang Y. Repair of meniscal defect using an induced myoblast-loaded polyglycolic acid mesh in a canine model. Experimental and Therapeutic Medicine. 2012;**3**:293-298

[173] Zorzi C, Rigotti S, Screpis D, Giordan N, Piovan G. A new hydrogel for the conservative treatment of meniscal lesions: A randomized controlled study. Joints. 2015;**3**:136-145

[174] Baek J, Sovani S, Glembotski NE, Du J, Jin S, Grogan SP, D'Lima DD. Repair of avascular meniscus tears with electrospun collagen scaffolds seeded with human cells. Tissue Engineering. Part A. 2016;**22**:436-448

[175] Li P, Zhang W, Yu H, Zheng L, Yang L, Liu G, Sheng C, Gui H, Ni S, Shi F. Applying electrospun gelatin/poly(lactic acid-co-glycolic acid) bilayered nanofibers to fabrication of meniscal tissue engineering scaffold. Journal of Nanoscience and Nanotechnology. 2016;**16**:4718-4726

[176] Martin JT, Milby AH, Ikuta K, Poudel S, Pfeifer CG, Elliott DM, Smith HE, Mauck RL. A radiopaque electrospun scaffold for engineering fibrous musculoskeletal tissues: Scaffold characterization and in vivo applications. Acta Biomaterialia. 2015;**26**:97-104

[177] Schwartz JA, Wang W, Goldstein T, Grande DA. Tissue engineered meniscus repair: Influence of cell passage number, tissue origin, and biomaterial carrier. Cartilage. 2014;**5**:165-171

[178] Shimomura K, Bean AC, Lin H, Nakamura N, Tuan RS. In vitro repair of meniscal radial tear using aligned electrospun nanofibrous scaffold. Tissue Engineering. Part A. 2015;**21**:2066-2075

[179] Oda S, Otsuki S, Kurokawa Y, Hoshiyama Y, Nakajima M, Neo M. A new method for meniscus repair using type I collagen scaffold and infrapatellar fat pad. Journal of Biomaterials Applications. 2015;**29**:1439-1448

[180] Kwak HS, Nam J, Lee JH, Kim HJ, Yoo JJ. Meniscal repair in vivo using human chondrocyte-seeded PLGA mesh scaffold pretreated with platelet-rich plasma. Journal of Tissue Engineering and Regenerative Medicine. 2014;**11**:471-480

[181] Dai Z, Li K, Chen Z, Liao Y, Yang L, Liu C, Ding W. Repair of avascular meniscal injuries using juvenile meniscal fragments: An in vitro organ culture study. Journal of Orthopaedic Research. 2013;**31**:1514-1519

[182] Freymann U, Endres M, Goldmann U, Sittinger M, Kaps C. Toward scaffold-based meniscus repair: Effect of human serum, hyaluronic acid and TGF-ss3 on cell recruitment and re-differentiation. Osteoarthritis and Cartilage. 2013;**21**:773-781

[183] Cucchiarini M, Schmidt K, Frisch J, Kohn D, Madry H. Promotes the healing of human meniscal lesions ex vivo on explanted menisci. The American Journal of Sports Medicine. 2015;**43**:1197-1205

[184] Zhang H, Leng P, Zhang J. Enhanced meniscal repair by overexpression of hIGF-1 in a full-thickness model. Clinical Orthopaedics and Related Research. 2009;**467**:3165-3174

[185] Zhang HN, Leng P, Wang YZ, Zhang J. Treating human meniscal fibrochondrocytes with hIGF-1 gene by liposome. Clinical Orthopaedics and Related Research. 2009;**467**:3175-3182

[186] Forriol F, Longo UG, Duart J, Ripalda P, Vaquero J, Loppini M, Romeo G, Campi S, Khan WS, Muda AO, Denaro V. VEGF, BMP-7, Matrigel(TM), hyaluronic acid, in vitro cultured chondrocytes and trephination for healing of the avascular portion of the meniscus. An experimental study in sheep. Current Stem Cell Research & Therapy. 2014;**10**:69-76

[187] Kawanishi Y, Nakasa T, Shoji T, Hamanishi M, Shimizu R, Kamei N, Usman MA, Ochi M. Intra-articular injection of synthetic microRNA-210 accelerates avascular meniscal healing in rat medial meniscal injured model. Arthritis Research & Therapy. 2014;**16**:488

[188] He W, Liu YJ, Wang ZG, Guo ZK, Wang MX, Wang N. Enhancement of meniscal repair in the avascular zone using connective tissue growth factor in a rabbit model. Chinese Medical Journal. 2011;**124**:3968-3975

[189] Freymann U, Endres M, Neumann K, Scholman HJ, Morawietz L, Kaps C. Expanded human meniscus-derived cells in 3-D polymer-hyaluronan scaffolds for meniscus repair. Acta Biomaterialia. 2012;**8**:677-685

[190] Lee HP, Kaul G, Cucchiarini M, Madry H. Nonviral gene transfer to human meniscal cells. Part I: Transfection analyses and cell transplantation to meniscus explants. International Orthopaedics. 2014;**38**:1923-1930

[191] Lee HP, Rey-Rico A, Cucchiarini M, Madry H. Nonviral gene transfer into human meniscal cells. Part II: Effect of three-dimensional environment and overexpression of human fibroblast growth factor 2. International Orthopaedics. 2014;**38**:1931-1936

[192] Narita A, Takahara M, Sato D, Ogino T, Fukushima S, Kimura Y, Tabata Y. Biodegradable gelatin hydrogels incorporating fibroblast growth factor 2 promote healing of horizontal tears in rabbit meniscus. Arthroscopy. 2012;**28**:255-263

[193] Pabbruwe MB, Kafienah W, Tarlton JF, Mistry S, Fox DJ, Hollander AP. Repair of meniscal cartilage white zone tears using a stem cell/collagen-scaffold implant. Biomaterials. 2010;**31**:2583-2591

[194] Kopf S, Birkenfeld F, Becker R, Petersen W, Starke C, Wruck CJ, Tohidnezhad M, Varoga D, Pufe T. Local treatment of meniscal lesions with vascular endothelial growth factor. The Journal of Bone and Joint Surgery. American Volume. 2010;**92**:2682-2691

[195] Riera KM, Rothfusz NE, Wilusz RE, Weinberg JB, Guilak F, McNulty AL. Interleukin-1, tumor necrosis factor-alpha, and transforming growth factor-beta 1 and integrative meniscal repair: Influences on meniscal cell

proliferation and migration. Arthritis Research & Therapy. 2011;**13**:R187

[196] Forriol F, Ripalda P, Duart J, Esparza R, Gortazar AR. Meniscal repair possibilities using bone morphogenetic protein-7. Injury. 2014;**45**(Suppl 4):S15-S21

[197] Kean CO, Brown RJ, Chapman J. The role of biomaterials in the treatment of meniscal tears. PeerJ. 2017;**5**:e4076

[198] Monibi FA, Cook JL. Tissue-derived extracellular matrix bioscaffolds: Emerging applications in cartilage and meniscus repair. Tissue Engineering. Part B, Reviews. 2017;**23**:386-398

[199] Numpaisal PO, Rothrauff BB, Gottardi R, Chien CL, Tuan RS. Rapidly dissociated autologous meniscus tissue enhances meniscus healing: An in vitro study. Connective Tissue Research. 2017;**58**:355-365

[200] Rey-Rico A, Cucchiarini M, Madry H. Hydrogels for precision meniscus tissue engineering: A comprehensive review. Connective Tissue Research. 2017;**58**:317-328

[201] Ishimura M, Ohgushi H, Habata T, Tamai S, Fujisawa Y. Arthroscopic meniscal repair using fibrin glue. Part II: Clinical applications. Arthroscopy. 1997;**13**:558-563

[202] Ishimura M, Ohgushi H, Habata T, Tamai S, Fujisawa Y. Arthroscopic meniscal repair using fibrin glue. Part I: Experimental study. Arthroscopy. 1997;**13**:551-557

[203] Patel S, Rodriguez-Merchan EC, Haddad FS. The use of fibrin glue in surgery of the knee. Journal of Bone and Joint Surgery. British Volume (London). 2010;**92**:1325-1331

[204] Graham LD, Danon SJ, Johnson G, Braybrook C, Hart NK, Varley RJ, Evans MD, McFarland GA, Tyler MJ, Werkmeister JA, Ramshaw JA. Biocompatibility and modification of the protein-based adhesive secreted by the Australian frog *Notaden bennetti*. Journal of Biomedical Materials Research. Part A. 2010;**93**:429-441

[205] Graham LD, Glattauer V, Huson MG, Maxwell JM, Knott RB, White JW, Vaughan PR, Peng Y, Tyler MJ, Werkmeister JA, Ramshaw JA. Characterization of a protein-based adhesive elastomer secreted by the Australian frog *Notaden bennetti*. Biomacromolecules. 2005;**6**:3300-3312

[206] Graham LD, Glattauer V, Li D, Tyler MJ, Ramshaw JA. The adhesive skin exudate of *Notaden bennetti* frogs (Anura: Limnodynastidae) has similarities to the prey capture glue of Euperipatoides sp. velvet worms (Onychophora: Peripatopsidae). Comparative Biochemistry and Physiology. Part B, Biochemistry & Molecular Biology. 2013;**165**:250-259

[207] Millar NL, Bradley TA, Walsh NA, Appleyard RC, Tyler MJ, Murrell GA. Frog glue enhances rotator cuff repair in a laboratory cadaveric model. Journal of Shoulder and Elbow Surgery. 2009;**18**:639-645

[208] Nowak R. Frog glue repairs damaged cartilage. New Scientist. 5 October 2004

[209] Szomor Z, Murrell GAC, Appleyard RC. Use of *Notaden bennetti* frog-glue for meniscal repair. Techniques in Knee Surgery. 2008;**7**:261-265

[210] Bochynska AI, Hannink G, Grijpma DW, Buma P. Tissue adhesives for meniscus tear repair: An overview of current advances and prospects for future clinical solutions. Journal of Materials Science. Materials in Medicine. 2016;**27**:85

[211] Bochynska AI, Van Tienen TG, Hannink G, Buma P, Grijpma

DW. Development of biodegradable hyper-branched tissue adhesives for the repair of meniscus tears. Acta Biomaterialia. 2016;**32**:1-9

[212] Brubaker CE, Messersmith PB. The present and future of biologically inspired adhesive interfaces and materials. Langmuir. 2012;**28**:2200-2205

[213] Shao H, Bachus KN, Stewart RJ. A water-borne adhesive modeled after the sandcastle glue of *P. californica*. Macromolecular Bioscience. 2009;**9**:464-471

[214] Simson JA, Strehin IA, Allen BW, Elisseeff JH. Bonding and fusion of meniscus fibrocartilage using a novel chondroitin sulfate bone marrow tissue adhesive. Tissue Engineering. Part A. 2013;**19**:1843-1851

[215] Kamimura T, Kimura M. Meniscal repair of degenerative horizontal cleavage tears using fibrin clots: Clinical and arthroscopic outcomes in 10 cases. Orthopaedic Journal of Sports Medicine. 2014;**2**:2325967114555678

[216] Guo J, Wang W, Hu J, Xie D, Gerhard E, Nisic M, Shan D, Qian G, Zheng S, Yang J. Synthesis and characterization of anti-bacterial and anti-fungal citrate-based mussel-inspired bioadhesives. Biomaterials. 2016;**85**:204-217

[217] Mehdizadeh M, Weng H, Gyawali D, Tang L, Yang J. Injectable citrate-based mussel-inspired tissue bioadhesives with high wet strength for sutureless wound closure. Biomaterials. 2012;**33**:7972-7983

[218] Weir C, Morel-Kopp MC, Gill A, Tinworth K, Ladd L, Hunyor SN, Ward C. Mesenchymal stem cells: Isolation, characterisation and in vivo fluorescent dye tracking. Heart, Lung & Circulation. 2008;**17**:395-403

[219] Tienen TG, Heijkants RG, de Groot JH, Schouten AJ, Pennings AJ, Veth RP, Buma P. Meniscal replacement in dogs. Tissue regeneration in two different materials with similar properties. Journal of Biomedical Materials Research Part B: Applied Biomaterials. 2006;**76**:389-396

[220] Wong CC, Kuo TF, Yang TL, Tsuang YH, Lin MF, Chang CH, Lin YH, Chan WP. Platelet-rich fibrin facilitates rabbit meniscal repair by promoting Meniscocytes proliferation, migration, and extracellular matrix synthesis. International Journal of Molecular Sciences. 2017;**18**. pii: E1722

[221] Chahla J, Kennedy NI, Geeslin AG, Moatshe G, Cinque ME, DePhillipo NN, LaPrade RF. Meniscal repair with fibrin clot augmentation. Arthroscopy Techniques. 2017;**6**:e2065-e2069

[222] Kowalski C, Gallo RA. Platelet-rich fibrin clot-augmented repair of horizontal cleavage meniscal tear. Arthroscopy Techniques. 2017;**6**:e2047-e2051

[223] Pan Z, Wu Y, Zhang X, Fu Q, Li J, Yang Y, Yu D, Xu Y, Lu X, Sun H, Heng BC, Bunpetch V, Zhang S, Ouyang H. Delivery of epidermal growth factor receptor inhibitor via a customized collagen scaffold promotes meniscal defect regeneration in a rabbit model. Acta Biomaterialia. 2017;**62**:210-221

[224] Zhang S, Matsushita T, Kuroda R, Nishida K, Matsuzaki T, Matsumoto T, Takayama K, Nagai K, Oka S, Tabata Y, Nagamune K, Kurosaka M. Local administration of simvastatin stimulates healing of an avascular meniscus in a rabbit model of a meniscal defect. The American Journal of Sports Medicine. 2016;**44**:1735-1743

[225] Bochynska AI, Hannink G, Verhoeven R, Grijpma DW, Buma P. The effect of tissue surface modification with collagenase and addition of TGF-beta3 on the healing potential of meniscal tears repaired with tissue glues in vitro. Journal of Materials Science. Materials in Medicine. 2017;**28**:22

Chapter 4

Bio-Engineered Meniscus for Tissue Engineering

Azran Azhim, Najian Ibrahim and Fatihah Yusof

Abstract

Meniscus plays fundamental roles in the knee mechanisms and functions. It acts as a shock absorber where it enables even distribution of forces, and also lubricates knee joints. Meniscal injuries could result to the onset of degenerative osteoarthritis if proper treatments are delayed. To date, treatment of meniscal injuries are more towards conservative methods and surgical approach commonly known as meniscectomy. Attempts to develop scaffolds for meniscus implants from synthetic and biological sources have been done in the recent years. This approach involves a multidisciplinary study known as tissue engineering and regenerative medicine. It involves the combination of three crucial aspects; the choice of chondrogenic/stem cells, bioscaffolds and favourable environmental factors such as growth factors. This chapter discusses and highlights on the currently available meniscal scaffolds that have been explored before. Focus is also directed on the potential of decellularized extracellular matrix (ECM), prepared through sonication treatment that produced scaffolds which mimics natural meniscus. The evaluation of decellularized scaffolds was portrayed through recellularization using cells namely chondrocytes, fibrochondrocytes and stem cells in order to regenerate new functional tissue. In short, this chapter serves as a representation of current approaches aiming in bio-engineering the meniscal scaffolds as meniscus tissue replacement.

Keywords: meniscus, bioscaffolds, decellularization, recellularization, implant

1. Introduction

Tissue engineering is deemed as a promising therapeutic tool in treating disease and injuries. There are three crucial aspects in determining the success of this approach which is by combining cells, biomaterial scaffolds and biologically active molecules such as growth factors. Developing three-dimensional scaffolds or constructs that could serve similarly as native tissue is utterly important. A scaffold should provide support and space for cells to grow, migrate and adhere and continually retain their phenotype. Hence, scaffolds should be biocompatible and biodegradable in the sense that it is able to propagate appropriate signals for the seeded cells execute normal cell homeostasis and processes.

Specifically, numerous growth factors have been used on meniscal fibrochondrocytes to evaluate their potential in healing tears or on protein synthesis using cell culture conditions. The most utilized is transforming growth factor-*b* (TGF-*b*). Studies by Marx et al. and Dunsmore et al. showed that TGF-*b* increases the proteoglycan synthesis of fibrochondrocytes from all different sections of the meniscus. Besides, hepatocyte growth factor (HGF) or bone-morphogenic protein-2 (BMP-2) was also shown to increase DNA synthesis. To add, cell migration rate improved with the usage of HGF and BMP-2 [1, 2] Other growth factor such as interleukin-1 (IL-1) was also reported to stimulate migration of cells taken from the peripheral third of the tissue. The famous fibroblastic growth factor (FGF) was studies by Webber et al. to show proliferation and stimulate the growth of fibrochondrocytes and human platelet lysate (PL) [3].

Next, the key aspect in the success of tissue engineering is the development of effective scaffolds which can serve to replace injured or damaged tissue. Thus for a successful meniscus replacement, consideration in the optimal scaffolds properties such as biomechanical, immunogenicity and potential to recellularize cells are important to be scrutinized. The highlight of this chapter would be discoursing different options in developing novel scaffolds of meniscal tissue replacement. The meniscus primarily functions as a load bearer and shock absorber. Degenerative or traumatic loss of meniscal tissue sometimes requires multiple surgical procedures to be treated. Ideally, treatment of meniscal injury should be focusing on the preservation and restoration of the meniscus function. However, effort of complete replacement of meniscus is deemed warranted in more severe cases. Various types of transplant have been done at the experimental and clinical level for example allogenic and autologous meniscus transplant. Issues such as host reactions towards major histocompatibility complexes of the donor, lead to progressive decellularization and consecutive failure of the transplant in meniscus allograft transplantation. To date, none of the proposed replacement methods could provide long-term chondroprotective effect. Scaffolds are necessary for tissue engineered meniscus replacement and considerations such as biomechanical, cell toxicity and immunological response of the host towards the scaffolds are crucial to be scrutinized. There is evidence suggesting that degenerative tears in older patients without mechanical symptoms can be effectively treated non-operatively with a structured physical therapy programme as a first line. Even if these patients later require meniscectomy they will still achieve similar functional outcomes than if they had initially been treated surgically. While, partial meniscectomy is more suitable for symptomatic tears which is hard to repair but could still preserve meniscal function.

2. Composition and cell characteristics of meniscus

Meniscus possesses a highly heterogeneous extracellular matrix (ECM) and has a wide range of cell distribution [4]. The ECM of meniscus is categorized by region. Collagen type I accounts for >80% of the composition in the red-red region by dry weight, and the remaining content comprises <1%, including collagen types II, III, IV, VI, and XVIII [5]. There is about 70% of collagen from the dry weight in the white-white region. On the other hand, collagen types II and I account for 60 and 40%, respectively. Next, the cell population in meniscus is categorized into 4 types based on where it resides. First, the outer one-third of the meniscal area is comprised of fibroblast-like cells, demonstrated by elongated shapes while outer periphery contain many cell processes like fibroblasts. Second, the inner two-thirds of the meniscal region mainly contain fibrochondrocytes, oval to round in shape. The inner avascular region comprised more rounded and chondrocyte-like cells. Lastly, fusiform cells are positioned parallel to the meniscal surface at the superficial zone [6].

3. Currently available scaffolds for meniscus

Meniscus scaffolds serves as a platform for the ingrowth of cells and provide support for the remodeling of the native tissue. There are two categories of scaffolds available; synthetic and biological types. There is a wide variety of synthetic scaffolds that have been explored. Polymer based scaffolds have been tested in a few experimental animal studies. Fibrocartilage-like tissue was able to grow in about 3 months' time after the seeding/implantation [7]. They also reported that in control group, degeneration of hyaline cartilage proceeded slower but could not be halted. To add, other bioabsorbable synthetic polymers, such as polyurethane (PU), polyglycolic acid (PGA), polylactic acid, and poly (ε- caprolactone) (PCL) are also widely studies to play important part in supporting the development of meniscal scaffolds [8, 9]. The main advantages of using polymer as the main material in scaffolds development is that they provide versatility, comparable biomechanical properties with native tissues and easily available material supply. However, there are some downside of using synthetic polymers which include their hydrophobic properties, non-biocompatibility issues, immunorejection and inflammation. Thus, many attempts have been done to improve polymer based scaffolds. One of them is Koller et al. whom had attempt to enhance the bioactivity of synthetic scaffolds by adding polyethylene terephthalate (PET) to hyaluronic acid/PCL scaffolds and the results were positive [10]. Scaffolds with PET were recorded to express more type II collagen mRNA and secreted more GAGs than without PET. Besides that, Baker and Mauck developed aligned (AL) scaffolds by electrospinning whereby cells in the AL group showed AL morphology whereas those in the control group took a polygonal shape [11]. Koller et al. improved PGA by reinforcing bonding with PLGA at a ratio of 75:25 in order to fabricate meniscus-like scaffolds [10]. Allogenic meniscal cells were seeded into the scaffolds *in vitro* for 1 week to replace the medial meniscus in rabbits. The results showed neomenisci are able to be regenerated which is similar to the native meniscus. However, the newly form neomenisci were not capable to prevent articular cartilage from further degenerating.

They are two main types of natural scaffolds which are tissue derived materials, extra cellular matrix (ECM) components and decellularized tissue. Some of the tissue derived materials that have been studied comprised of small intestine submucosa (SIS), periosteal tissue, and perichondral tissue. Cook et al. have done studies of SIS in dogs and showed promising results. However the study only lasted for 12 week and no mechanical testing was done [12]. One of the significant tests is their major animal trial which consisted of removing 80% of the medial meniscus of the dog and replacing it with this scaffold. The results after 3 years of implantation were promising which showed no degeneration of the articular cartilage. Walsh and co-workers utilized periosteal tissue in rabbits, showed both hyaline cartilage and bone growing in the repair tissue at the end of the 24- week trial. The results from perichondral tissue were not much better; these 12-month sheep tests gave repair tissue that resembled the meniscus grossly, but the tensile modulus of the repair tissue was much lower than native menisci. Besides that, collagen based scaffolds have also been developed from porcine small intestine submucosa (SIS) but however they failed to portray consistent results in experimental animal studies [13, 14].

Next, naturally derived ECM components include collagen, proteoglycans and elastin molecules. These scaffolds were made from collagen retrieved from bovine tendons and then molded into a circumferential orientation. It is now is already in phase II clinical trials. Collagen scaffolds portrayed a more convincing result whereby Stone, Rodkey, and co-workers used collagen-GAG scaffolds [15].

Attempts in developing decellularized tissues while retaining its ECM properties have been recently studied. Simple tissues as well as complicated organs have been decellularized and decellularization methods have been optimized to completely remove the cellular components while keeping the ECM intact. ECM scaffolds and substrates are very ideal candidates for tissue engineering as it functions in providing supporting materials for cell regulations and functions such as cell survival, proliferation, morphogenesis and differentiation. By comparing these three types of scaffolds, it is undeniable to claim that decellularized based scaffolds which could still contain ECM properties hold the greatest potential in developing ideal scaffolds for meniscus. The next sub topic will be discussed trials to develop decellularized matrices various techniques; biological, chemical and physical methods.

4. Decellularized meniscal scaffolds

Decellularized scaffolds are expected to provide a better alternative for implant development in tissue engineering. Besides of it being a suitable microenvironment for cells, it also preserves appropriate meniscal geometry. Nevertheless, some challenges should be addressed to obtain ideal meniscal scaffolds. Because of meniscus natural shape, it will make it tougher for cells to evenly penetrate a decellularized meniscus. Not only that, an abundance of bone morphogenetic protein-2 (BMP-2), a member of the TGF-β superfamily will directly stimulate MSC differentiation and can affect cell migration [16]. A study by Minehara et al. used recombinant human bone morphogenetic protein-2 (rhBMP-2) loading in solvent-preserved human menisci to induce migration of chondrocytes into decellularized which successfully induces migration of chondrocytes thus improving proteoglycan production *in vitro* [17]. Thus, decellularized scaffolds face a challenge of allowing better cell penetration and migration which depends on variety kinds of exogenous chemokines.

One of the effective detergents used to decellularize menisci is SDS whereby collagen structure is retained [18]. Biomechanical testing using repetitive ball indentation test (stiffness, N/mm; residual force, N; relative compression force, N) on the processed tissue were similar to those of the intact meniscus, and the histological results showed no residual cells. Besides that, Maier et al. used a self-developed enzymatic process to treat ovine menisci whereby results suggested that native cells and immunogenic proteins (MHC-1/MHC-2) are completely removed while retaining significant biomechanical traits [19]. On the other side, Stabile et al. attempted to improve the porosity of decellularized scaffolds by applying concomitant decellularization and oxidation processes [20]. Azhim et al. implemented neoteric sonication decellularization system to produce decellularized bovine meniscal scaffolds [21]. These scaffolds provide similar biomechanical properties of native meniscus, and were able to completely remove the immunogenic cell components. However, the sonication treatment compromised the native ECM components and collagen fiber arrangement. Thus, using decellularized scaffolds are great alternative for implants but more improvising needs to be done in order for successful integration into patients.

5. Decellularization strategies

Biological scaffolds had been widely used in tissue engineering and regenerative medicine field because it virtually resembles native tissue due to the presence of versatile bioactive nature within the extracellular matrix components [22]. The preparation of natural biological scaffolds involves a process known as decellularization as shown in **Figure 1**. Decellularization is a process that removes whole cellular components within the existing tissue while preserving the composition, integrity and mechanics of the three dimensional extracellular matrix scaffolds to the extent possible [23, 24]. The elimination of the antigens and cellular components from the tissue-derived scaffolds able to reduce the potential immune rejection and inflammation from occurring [25]. The choice of decellularization method varies depending on the characteristics of the particular tissues itself such as geometric considerations, cells and matrix density [26, 18]. An effective and ideal decellularization process supposedly manages to balance the removal of cellular components and preservation of matrix. There are various techniques that had been developed to obtain the most effective outcomes for fabrication of meniscus bioscaffolds using decellularization process. According to Chen & Kawazoe and Gilbert, to obtain an effective decellularization effect, it is encouraged for the method to be applied in combination [22, 26].

Three main strategies had been performed comprised of biological, chemicals and physical methods. For biological method, it is based on treatments using the enzymes such as proteases (trypsin, dispase), nucleases (DNase & RNase), collagenase, lipase and others [23, 27]. Enzymes are known as substances that have high specificity onto biological substrate which able to cleave or hydrolyze the particular bonds within the tissue structure during decellularization. According to Badylak et al. enzymatic decellularization treatment need a long treatment time and has difficulty to achieve complete cellular components removal alone [28]. Moreover, an extensive treatment time up to 2 days will affecting the ECM ultrastructure components, thus weakening the mechanical properties of the tissues. A study done by Maier et al. treated ovine meniscus with trypsin, collagenase and protease enzyme had successfully decellularized the tissue but with GAGs destruction [19].

The second option is the chemical methods which are further expanded into acid & based treatments, alcohols and also surfactants. According to Seiichi et al., chemical detergents treatment was investigated to be the most commonly used for decellularization technique [29]. The mechanism of acid& bases in decellularizing tissues is by catalyzing hydrolytic degradation of the biomolecules that able to dissociate the DNA from the ECM and disrupting nucleic acid [23, 30]. Chen et al. had performed a decellularization of porcine meniscus using five types of acid consist of acetic acid, formic acid, peracetic acid, succinic acid, malic acid and citric acid with different acid immersion incubation time of 2, 4, 6, 8, 10 and 12 hours [31]. The results portrayed that formic acid with 2 h immersion treatment is the most

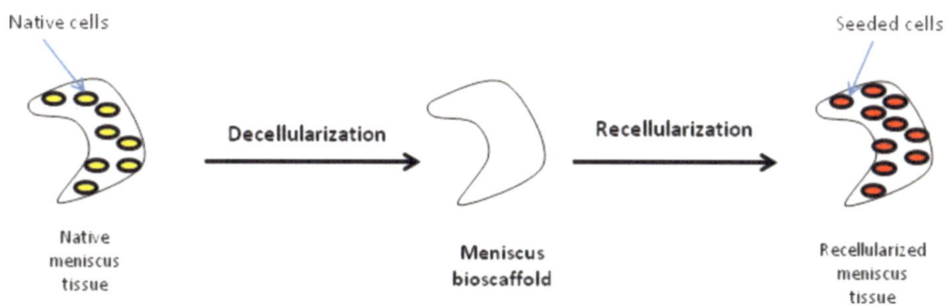

Figure 1.
Decellularization and recellularization of meniscus tissue.

effective because it managed to remove almost 96% of the DNA contents with minor adverse effect on ECM collagens and GAGs [31].

Various types of surfactants widely available for decellularization known as ionic, nonionic and zwitterionic detergents. Ionic detergent is recognized as the strongest acting detergent compared to others which are the most broadly applied in decellularization process [27, 32]. Sodium dodecyl sulfate (SDS), Triton X-200 and sodium deoxycholate are the examples of ionic detergents which are the commonly used for various types of tissue. In 2009, Sandmann et al. investigated and published a study on the effect of 2% SDS with 2 weeks incubation time onto biomechanical strength of human meniscus tissues [33]. It was proven that 2% SDS achieved complete cells removal with minor negative impacts on the biomechanical properties of prepared decellularized human meniscus.

Biological and chemical treatments might result in residual toxicity within the tissues, thus physical treatment for decellularization had been developed. Physical treatments involve freeze–thaw, high hydrostatic pressure, agitation and sonication to disrupt cell membranes and release the cellular components. High hydrostatic pressure system decellularized the tissue by applying pressure from specialized equipment that lead to high cost requirement. This system able to decellularize the tissue in short treatment time but have high risk of extracellular matrix (ECM) ultrastructure disruption due to baric formation of ice crystals throughout the process [34].

In 2010, a novel sonication decellularization with open system had been developed as a new candidate categorized under physical treatment. Sonication system utilizes the ultrasound power assisted by sodium dodecyl sulfate (SDS) to maximize the decellularization efficiency. Researchers and expertise have used ultrasound technology in a wide range of activities such as electrochemistry, food technology, chemical synthesis, material extraction, nanotechnology and surface cleaning [35]. Recently, the application of ultrasound is said to be one of the popular method for cell disruption, emulsification and homogenizing of biological matter [36]. The potential of ultrasound has lead to the development of sonication treatment.

Since 2010, a pilot study had been started by using aorta [21, 38–42] and meniscus tissues [21, 37, 43, 44] as model by testing using different sonication frequency and different percentage of SDS solution concentration that suit with the characteristics of the tissue [21, 37–41]. As for decellularized meniscus tissue preparation, primary study was done using 20 kHz frequency with 2% SDS solution for 10 hours treatment time that resulted in highest cells removal but there was minor presence of cells observed [37]. Thus, further study was done by increasing the sonication to 40 kHz frequency while minimizing the SDS concentration to 0.1% in order to preserve the bioscaffolds properties [21]. This study compared the sonication treated tissue with immersion treatment as control and native tissue. Based on the result of van Gieson staining portrayed in **Figure 2**, it revealed the complete cells removal from meniscus tissue by sonication system (C) where there is no nuclei stained can be observed compared to control (B) and native (A).

In 2014, Azhim et al. had developed a novel closed sonication decellularization system as shown in **Figure 3**. The ultrasonic transducer is the source of sonication that has three different set of frequency of 40, 120 and 170 kHz. The decellularization efficiency of sonication system was contributed mainly by sonication and also SDS detergent. Firstly, sonication influences the process by the disruption of the cell membrane and cell contents release by its phenomenon of acoustic cavitation. Besides that, sonication also assists the flow of SDS solution that thoroughly penetrates

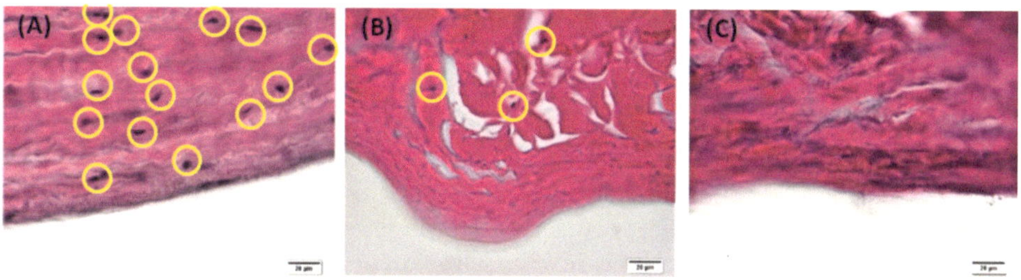

Figure 2.
Photographs of van Gieson staining from surface part of native tissue (A), immersion treated tissue (B), sonication treated tissue (C) with 40× magnification. Yellow circle demonstrated the dark blue nuclei stained [21].

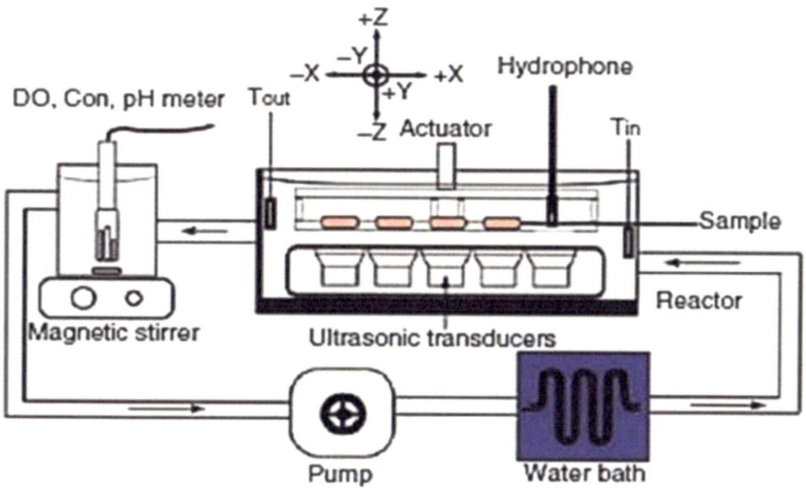

Figure 3.
Sonication decellularization system consists of ultrasonic transducers, pump, cooling water bath, reactor, actuator, temperature monitor, hydrophone, and multiparameter meter that consists of dissolved oxygen (DO), conductivity and pH sensor [39].

within tissue sample. Ionic SDS detergents aid in decellularization by solubilizing nuclear cellular membranes and removing cells residues from the tissue specimens.

6. Recellularization strategies for regeneration of engineered meniscus

In tissue engineering and regenerative medicine, the preparation of engineered meniscus tissue required triad components comprised of scaffolds, cells and growth factors. Basically, the cells will be recellularized onto artificial or natural biological scaffolds with the presence of growth factors for regeneration of tissue. Recellularization using the three dimensional decellularized scaffolds had been one of the attention recently because it resembles natural tissue that have similar biological compositions of the ECM. It is therefore an advantage for the decellularized scaffolds to provide a better environment for the adhesion, differentiation and proliferation of the seeded cells to regenerate functional tissues [45, 46].

According to Chen, recellularization is a crucial part in tissue engineering where cell-seeded constructs can be prepared [31]. This constructs are believed to have many potential advantages for in vitro and in vivo study. First and foremost, it manages to provide specific microenvironment for cells to proliferate and perform cellular activities for production of ECM. Besides that, cell seeded constructs also ease the integration between scaffolds and native tissues once implanted into the recipient [31].

The advancements of tissue engineering nowadays had the potential to drive meniscus regeneration into clinically relevant strategies and as a promising avenue to improve meniscus repair. For meniscus tissue engineering, various types of cell sources currently being utilized for recellularization process to prepare the cell seeded constructs [47–49]. Different types of cells stimulate different outcome. Ideal cells that suitable for recellularization of meniscus scaffolds should be easy to obtain, low immunogenicity level and able to regenerate the ECM components within the tissue [7]. In this chapter, we will give an overview of promising cell sources that hold great potential meniscus tissue regeneration. There are two main classifications of promising cells available for seeding processes which are stem cells/progenitor cells and mature cells. **Table 1** summarizes the cell sources that are available and broadly applied in meniscus tissue engineering.

6.1 Stem cells/progenitor cells

Stem cells are known as undifferentiated cells that able to proliferate and differentiate into many specialized cell types. Two main characteristics of stem cells that distinguish them with other cells is that stem cells are multipotent where it can be induced into specific tissue with specific functions and it has long term self-renewal [50, 51]. Mesenchymal stem cells are the most studied stem cells that can be harvested from several musculoskeletal tissues such as bone, bone marrow, adipose tissue, synovial membrane and cartilage [47, 52]. Drawbacks of using mesenchymal stem cells lies in the complex understanding of required stimuli to direct the differentiation process to a desired lineage [48]. Besides that, once the microenvironment changes and undergo hypertrophy, the differentiated phenotype can be easily lost [53].

Bone marrow mesenchymal stem cells (BM-MSCs) derived from bone marrow compartment with high proliferative activity is identified as heterogeneous population of stem cells capable to undergo self-renewal [54]. The extraction of BM-MSCs is quit complex because need to undergo bone marrow aspiration procedure which is invasive. BM-MSCs have the ability to differentiate into three lineages of skeletal tissue cells in appropriate in vitro condition; osteoblasts, adipocytes and chondrocytes [55]. Few studies had been attempted in meniscus tissue engineering using BM-MSCs. An in vitro study performed by Yamasaki et al., 2×10^5 cells were seeded onto decellularized rat meniscus in 48 well plate, incubated for 1, 2 and 4 weeks the cell-scaffolds constructs were evaluated with few analyses [56]. The results obtained from the analyses revealed that there was sufficient repopulation of BM-MSCs within the scaffolds. It was noted that there was sufficient generation of ECM compositions such as collagen and GAGs over 4 weeks in culture that resembles the content in control group. Evaluation of mechanical integrity for regenerated tissues portrayed similar stiffness with normal meniscus tissue after incubated 2 weeks in vitro culture. Unfortunately, this study lack of in vivo study which will be done in further study.

Adipose stem cells (ASCs) are considered as alternative cell sources that available in emerging tissue regeneration. This ASCs was discovered in the early 2000 that have high self-renewal capacity and capable to differentiate into three different cell lineages known as adipocytes, osteoblast and chondrocytes if subjected to desired stimuli [47]. It was reported that the isolation of ASCs is easier compared to BM-MSc that are commonly isolated from the intrapatellar fat pad of the knee and is not invasive. [57, 58]. An in vitro study using adipose mesenchymal stem

Classification of cells	Type of cells	Results	References
Stem cells/ progenitor cells	Bone-marrow (BM)-derived MSCs	Extracellular matrices was successfully synthesized at early phase with adequate stiffness observed after 2 weeks culture.	[56]
	Synovium MSCs	Early phase of synovial coverage on injured area was induced and promoted meniscus regeneration	[61]
	Adipose stem cells (ASCs)	Managed to partially formed meniscus-like tissue with no detectable amount of GAG	[59]
	Cartilage progenitor cells (CPCs)	Cells migrated to the tears injury site while promoting bridging across the site	[64]
	Myoblast	High cell yield, rapid proliferation activity with similar biochemical compositions compared to control	[66]
	Articular chondrocytes	Cells proliferated and synthesized ECM production (collagen & gag)	[68]
		High proliferation rates and the tissue generated had notable amount of GAG and collagen type II	[66]
		Cells infiltrated rapidly and distributed evenly in vitro and in vivo at Day 14	[69]
		Chondrocytes able to synthesized meniscal tissue in an *in vivo* situation	[69]
Mature cells	Fibrochondrocytes	Cells survived and proliferated for over 28 days, demonstrating the feasibility of culturing cells within ECM scaffolds	[70]
		The cells manages to self assemble and produced ECM matrix of collagen type I and proteoglycans	[71]
	Fibroblasts	Fibroblastic cell morphology attached and infiltrated into the surface of scaffolds	[75]

Table 1.
Cells sources for meniscus tissues regeneration.

cells seeded on four types of different scaffolds incubated for 3 days had been accomplished by Moradi et al. in 2017 [59]. The cell seeded scaffolds were evaluated for mechanical integrity, biocompatibility and gene expression. The performed real time PCR after 3 weeks culture concluded that ASCs scaffolds had an increase in aggrecan and collagen type II expression compared to control group. For in vivo study, the ASCs scaffolds were implanted into rabbit model for 7 months to discover neomeniscus tissue formation. It was resulted that ASCs scaffolds were found to generate homogenous neomeniscus with poor quality [59].

In 2001, a study conducted by De Bari et al. that characterized the synovial MSCs reported that the cells capable to proliferate extensively and maintained their multilineage differentiation potential in vitro culture [60]. According to Ozeki et al., his study chose synovium MSCs to be seeded onto tendon grafts and assessed the meniscus regeneration through in vitro and in vivo. It was revealed that the tendon grafts with synovial MSCs succeeded to induce early phase of synovial coverage at the defect site and had better integration with the meniscus defect that promote meniscus regeneration compared to control group [61].

Recently, cartilage progenitor cells (CPCs) represented as new and potential great cell sources available for cartilage and meniscus tissue regeneration. CPCs are basically obtained from the full thickness of mature cartilage. The chondrocytes population was first isolated and need to further undergo differential adhesion to fibronectin process in order to obtain the CPCs [47, 62]. It was identified that CPCs appeared in fibrochondrocytes-like appearance with chondrogenic potential. These CPCs were reviewed to be resistant towards common problems faced by MSCs recognized as terminal differentiation and also hypertrophy [47, 63]. Hypertrophy is a situation where the cells tend to enlarge with increase in cell mass that required more energy [63]. According to Williams, CPSs were reported to experience better complex chondrogenesis processes compared to other mesenchymal stem cells [62]. CPCs supplied onto meniscus with tears demonstrated that the cells capable to migrate to the tears site of tears injury while promoting bridging across the site [64]. Unfortunately, the study about CPCS in meniscus tissue engineering is still limited.

Myoblasts are considered as adult stem cells candidate that have multiple differentiation potentials that capable to differentiate mainly into myocytes, adipocytes and osteocytes [65]. Myoblasts were recognized as easily accessed cells with relatively abundant availability with acute donor site morbidity [66, 67]. Chondrogenic differentiation of myoblasts within PLGA scaffolds was concluded to have high cell yields with rapid cells proliferation. Besides that, it was observed that the biochemical compositions and mechanical strength of the implanted myoblast-scaffolds was similar to native tissue [66].

6.2 Mature cells

Mature cells are a nonprogenitor cells including chondrocytes, fibrochondrocytes and fibroblasts able to be derived from cartilage, meniscus and dermal tissues. The application of mature cells somehow managed to overcome major limitation of stem cells that mainly facing the hypertrophy occurrence [47].

As for articular chondrocytes (AC), it is principally derived from articular cartilage and can enzymatically isolate. A recent study was done where chondrocytes were seeded directly onto the layer of decellularized porcine meniscus and incubated for up to 28 days. It was reported that the cells able to proliferate healthily and synthesized the extracellular matrix such as collagen type II and GAG within the scaffolds [68]. Besides that, according to an analysis done by Marsano et al. that seeded the cells onto 3D pellet culture to investigate the growth and post-expansion chondrogenic capacity of chondrocytes [67]. Based on the evaluation done after pellet culture for 2, 4 and 6 weeks, it was indicated that articular chondrocytes resulted in high proliferation rate. This AC generated tissue was found to form abundant GAG and collagen type II in inner avascular region at the same time produced collagen type IV in outer vascular region [67]. There had been two other studies portrayed in **Table 1** that recellularized scaffolds with chondrocytes for meniscus regeneration [69, 70].

Meniscal fibrochondrocytes are investigated as one of the cell sources for meniscus regeneration which can be extracted easily from meniscus [19, 71]. Fibrochondrocytes distributed in all regions of meniscus but dominates more in the vascular outer layer that mainly composed of Type I collagen. The multilineage differentiation particularly favors more towards chondrogenesis and adipogenesis [72]. A study done by Maier et al. 2007 had successfully seeded the fibrochondrocytes onto the decellularized ovine meniscus. The results showed that the cells managed to infiltrate, survive and proliferate for more than 28 days in the scaffolds [19].

The red-red region of the meniscus that mainly exhibit collagen type II consist of fibroblast-like cells with elongated morphology [73]. This kind of cells frequently derived from reliable sources such as dermal skin that obtained from different body sites and also meniscus tissues. Fibroblasts play important roles in physiological process essentially in ECM production, inflammation and wound healing regulation [74]. Stapleton et al. had constructed decellularized scaffolds using freeze thaw method and Sodium dodecyl sulfate (SDS) detergent [75]. The prepared scaffolds were utilized for recellularization process using dermal fibroblasts cells for 7 days and proceed with implantation in GTKO mice. Based on the evaluation after 7 days of culture in decellularized meniscus, the fibroblasts successfully infiltrate the scaffolds to a depth of 150 mm and the cells were found to appear on the surface with flattened morphology [75].

7. Future prospects for meniscal tissue engineering

There is a dearth in the number of studies done currently in engineering meniscus as compared to other tissues like articular cartilage. The fundamental knowledge on meniscus and its mechanism needs to be fully understood for researchers and clinicians to target a problem. Besides that, knowledge fibrochondrocytes, chondrocytes and other mesenchymal stem cells reactions to a variety of growth factors need to be understood through a variety of tests, both from tissue engineering studies and meniscal repair enhancement studies. Meniscus scaffolds for future application should focus on engineering the entire functional unit which includes meniscal body with anterior and posterior ligaments. Great perception regarding the characteristics of the meniscus constructs in designing for meniscal replacement is important to the overall function. However, an intensive attempt in discovering the appropriate seed cells, biological and mechanical strength stimulation should be given more attention. Broad study on cell sources chose for recellularization should focusing more to in vivo study in animal model. The well performance of in vivo study might depend on several factors such as the quality of neotissue formed during in vitro. More importantly, the fabrication of engineered meniscus tissue with excellent mechanical strength and function that mimic native tissue is the key issue in this field. Good mechanical strength contributes to normal meniscus function. Besides that, three-dimensional construct printing could profit the development of meniscal scaffolds ideally. In short, the development bio-engineering ideal scaffolds for meniscal tissue engineering applications depend on the ability to preserve the biomechanical and biochemical properties of the tissue. The scaffolds should be biocompatible and emit minimum inflammatory effect on to the host.

Author details

Azran Azhim*, Najian Ibrahim and Fatihah Yusof
Department of Biomedical Sciences, Kulliyyah of Allied Health Sciences, International Islamic University Malaysia (IIUM), Jalan Sultan Ahmad Shah, Bandar Indera Mahkota, Kuantan, Pahang, Malaysia

*Address all correspondence to: azr2020@gmail.com

References

[1] Marx RE, Carlson ER, Eichstaedt RM, Schimmele SR, Strauss JE, Georgeff KR. Platelet-rich plasma: Growth factor enhancement for bone grafts. Oral Surgery, Oral Medicine, Oral Pathology, Oral Radiology, and Endodontology. 1998;**85**(6):638-646

[2] Dunsmore SE, Rubin JS, Kovacs SO, Chedid M, Parks WC, Welgus HG. Mechanisms of hepatocyte growth factor stimulation of keratinocyte metalloproteinase production. Journal of Biological Chemistry. 1996;**271**(40):24576-24582

[3] Webber CA, Chen YY, Hehr CL, Johnston J, McFarlane S. Multiple signaling pathways regulate FGF-2-induced retinal ganglion cell neurite extension and growth cone guidance. Molecular and Cellular Neuroscience. 2005;**30**(1):37-47

[4] Ahluwalia S, Fehm M, Murray MM, Martin SD, Spector M. Distribution of smooth muscle actin-containing cells in the human meniscus. Journal of Orthopaedic Research. 2001;**19**(4):659-664

[5] Moran CJ, Atmaca S, Declercq HA, Cornelissen MJ, Verdonk PC. Cell distribution and regenerative activity following meniscus replacement. International Orthopaedics. 2014;**38**(9):1937-1944

[6] Ahluwalia S, Fehm M, Murray MM, Martin SD, Spector M. Distribution of smooth muscle actin-containing cells in the human meniscus. Journal of Orthopaedic Research. 2001;**19**(4):659-664

[7] Cheung HY, Lau KT, Lu TP, Hui D. A critical review on polymer-based bio-engineered materials for scaffold development. Composites Part B: Engineering. 2007;**38**(3): 291-300

[8] Gloria A, De Santis R, Ambrosio L. Polymer-based composite scaffolds for tissue engineering. Journal of Applied Biomaterials & Biomechanics. 2010;**8**(2):57-67

[9] Gunatillake PA, Adhikari R. Biodegradable synthetic polymers for tissue engineering. European Cells & Materials. 2003;**5**(1):1-6

[10] Koller U, Nehrer S, Vavken P, Kapeller B, Windhager R, Chiari C. Polyethylene terephthalate (PET) enhances chondrogenic differentiation of ovine meniscocytes in a hyaluronic acid/polycaprolactone scaffold in vitro. International Orthopaedics. 2012;**36**(9):1953-1960

[11] Baker BM, Mauck RL. The effect of nanofiber alignment on the maturation of engineered meniscus constructs. Biomaterials. 2007;**28**(11):1967-1977

[12] Cook JL, Fox DB, Malaviya P, Tomlinson JL, Kuroki K, Cook CR, et al. Long-term outcome for large meniscal defects treated with small intestinal submucosa in a dog model. The American Journal of Sports Medicine. 2006;**34**(1):32-42

[13] Cook JL, Tomlinson JL, Arnoczky SP, Fox DB, Cook CR, Kreeger JM. Kinetic study of the replacement of porcine small intestinal submucosa grafts and the regeneration of meniscal-like tissue in large avascular meniscal defects in dogs. Tissue Engineering. 2001;**7**(3):321-334

[14] Fox DB, Cook JL, Arnoczky SP, Tomlinson JL, Kuroki K, Kreeger JM, et al. Fibrochondrogenesis of free intraarticular small intestinal submucosa scaffolds. Tissue Engineering. 2004;**10**(1-2):129-137

[15] Stone KR, Steadman JR, Rodkey WG, Li ST. Regeneration of meniscal cartilage with use of a collagen scaffold.

Analysis of preliminary data. The Journal of Bone and Joint Surgery. 1997;**79**(12):1770-1777

[16] Lieberman JR, Daluiski A, Einhorn TA. The role of growth factors in the repair of bone: Biology and clinical applications. The Journal of Bone and Joint Surgery. 2002;**84**(6):1032-1044

[17] Minehara H, Urabe K, Naruse K. A new technique for seeding chondrocytes onto solvent-preserved human meniscus using the chemokinetic effect of recombinant human bone morphogenetic protein-2. Cell and Tissue Banking. 2011;**12**(3):199-207

[18] Gilbert TW, Sellaro TL, Badylak SF. Decellularization of tissues and organs. Biomaterials. 2006;**27**(19):3675-3683

[19] Maier D, Braeun K, Steinhauser E, Ueblacker P, Oberst M, Kreuz PC, et al. In vitro analysis of an allogenic scaffold for tissue-engineered meniscus replacement. Journal of Orthopedic Research. 2007;**25**:1598-1608

[20] Stabile KJ, Odom D, Smith TL. An acellular, allograft-derived meniscus scaffold in an ovine model. Arthroscopy. 2010;**26**(7):936-948

[21] Azhim A, Ono T, Fukui Y, Morimoto Y, Furukawa K, Ushida T. Preparation of decellularized meniscal scaffolds using sonication treatment for tissue engineering. In: Proceedings of the 35th Annual International Conference of the IEEE Engineering in Medicine and Biology Society (EMBC '13); 3-7 July 2013. Osaka, Japan: IEEE; 2013. pp. 6953-6956

[22] Chen G, Kawazoe N. Decellularization techniques for tissue engineering. In: Encyclopedia of Analytical Chemistry. USA: John Wiley & Sons, Ltd; 2015. DOI: 10.1002/9780470027318.a9472

[23] Crapo PM, Gilbert TW, Badylak SF. An overview of tissue and whole organ decellularization processes. Biomaterials. 2011;**32**(12):3233-3243. DOI: 10.1016/j.biomaterials.2011.01.057

[24] Nakamura N, Kimura T, Kishida A. Overview of the development, applications, and future perspectives of decellularized tissues and organs. ACS Biomaterials Science & Engineering. 2017;**3**:1236-1244. DOI: 10.1021/acsbiomaterials.6b00506

[25] Patnaik SS, Wang B, Weed B, Werthheim JA, Liao J. Decellularized scaffolds: Concepts, methodologies, and applications in cardiac tissue engineering and whole-organ regeneration. In: Liu Q, editor. Tissue Regeneration: Where Nano-Structure Meets Biology. Singapore: World Scientific Company; 2003. pp. 1-48

[26] Keane TJ, Swinehart I, Badylak SF. Methods of tissue decellularization used for preparation of biologic scaffolds and in vivo relevance. Methods. 2015;**84**:25-34. DOI: 10.1016/j.ymeth.2015.03.005

[27] Gilpin A, Yang Y. Decellularization strategies for regenerative medicine: From processing techniques to applications. BioMed Research International. 2017:1-13. DOI: 10.1155/2017/9831534

[28] Badylak SF, Freytes DO, Gilbert TW. Extracellular matrix as a biological scaffold material: Structure and function. Acta Biomaterialia. 2009;**5**(1):1-13. DOI: 10.1016/j.actbio.2008.09.013

[29] Seiichi F, Kwangwoo N, Tsuyoshi K, Ayako M, Yoshihide H, Kazuo N, et al. The use of high-hydrostatic pressure treatment to decellularize blood vessels. Biomaterials. 2010;**31**(13):3590-3595. DOI: 10.1016/j.biomaterials.2010.01.073

[30] Gupta SK, Mishra NC. Decellularization methods for

scaffold fabrication. Methods in Molecular Biology. 2017:1-10. DOI: 10.1007/7651_2017_34

[31] Chen Y, Chen J, Zhang Z, Lou K, Zhang Q, Wang S, et al. Current advances in the development of natural meniscus scaffolds: Innovative approaches to decellularization and recellularization. Cell and Tissue Research. 2017;**370**(1):41-52. DOI: 10.1007/s00441-017-2605-0

[32] Haykal S, Soleas JP, Salna M, Hofer SO, Waddell TK. Determining the in vitro and in vivo immune response towards decellularized and recellularized porcine tracheal allografts for airway transplantation. Plastic and Reconstructive Surgery. 2013;**131**(5S):74

[33] Sandmann GH, Eichhorn S, Vogt S, Adamczyk C, Aryee S, Hoberg M, et al. Generation and characterization of a human acellular meniscus scaffold for tissue engineering. Journal of Biomedical Materials Research. 2008;**91A**(2):567-574. DOI: 10.1002/jbm.a.32269

[34] Borges EN, Silva RC, Futino DO, Rocha-Junior CMC, Amorim CA, Bao SN. Cryopreservation of swine ovarian tissue: Effect of different cryoprotectants on the structural preservation of preantral follicle oocytes. Cryobiology. 2009;**5**:195-200

[35] Chemart F, E-Huma Z, Khan KM. Applications of ultrasound in food technology: Processing, preservation and extraction. Ultrasonics Sonochemistry. 2011;**18**:813-835

[36] Saranya N, Devi P, Nithiyanantham S, Jeyalaxmi R. Cells disruption by ultrasonication. BioNanoScience. 2014;**4**(3):1-3

[37] Azhim A, Takahashi T, Muramatsu K, Morimoto Y, Tanaka M. Decellularization of meniscal tissue using ultrasound chemical process for tissue-engineered scaffold applications. In: 6th World Congress of Biomechanics (WCB 2010). Singapore: Springer Berlin Heidelberg; August 1-6, 2010. pp. 915-918

[38] Azhim A, Yamagami K, Muramatsu K, Morimoto Y, Tanaka M. The use of sonication treatment to completely decellularize blood arteries: A pilot study. In: Proceeding of IEEE Engineering in Medicine Biology Society; 30 August-3 September 2011; Boston, USA. pp. 2468-2471

[39] Azhim A, Shafiq M, Rasyada AR, Furukawa K, Ushida T. The impact of acoustic intensity on solution parameters and decellularization using sonication treatment. Journal of Biomaterial Tissue Engineering. 2015;**5**(3):195-203. DOI: 10.1166/jbt.2015.1300

[40] Azhim A, Yamagami K, Muramatsu K, Morimoto Y, Tanaka M, Furukawa KS, et al. The use of sonication treatment to completely decellularize aorta tissue. In: World Congress on Medical Physics and Biomedical Engineering, IFMBE Proceedings; 26-31 May 2012; Beijing, China. pp. 1987-1990

[41] Azhim A, Syazwani N, Morimoto Y, Furukawa KS, Ushida T. The use of sonication treatment to decellularize aortic tissues for preparation of bioscaffolds. Journal of Biomaterials Applications. 2014;**29**(1):130-141

[42] Syazwani N, Azhim A, Morimoto Y, Furukawa K, Ushida T. Decellularization of aorta tissue using sonication treatment as potential scaffold for vascular tissue engineering. Journal of Medical and Biological Engineering. 2015;**35**(2):258-269

[43] Norzarini A, Azhim A, Ushida T. Decellularized bovine meniscus in

morphological assessment prior to bioscaffold preparation, 10th Asian Control Conference; 31 May- 3 June 2015; Kota Kinabalu, Malaysia. pp. 1-4

[44] Norzarini A, Azhim A, Kitajima T, Feng Z, Sha'ban M. Characterization based on biomechanical properties for meniscus scaffolds by sonication decellularization treatment. Journal of Biomaterial Tissue Engineering. 2016;**7**(3):223-232

[45] Barkan D, Green JE, Chambers AF. Extracellular matrix: A gatekeeper in the transition from dormancy to metastatic growth. European Journal of Cancer. 2010;**46**(7):1181-1188. DOI: 10.1016/j.ejca.2010.02.027

[46] Tien J, Nelson CM. Microstructured extracellular matrices in tissue engineering and development: An update. Annals of Biomedical Engineering. 2014;**42**(7):1413-1423. DOI: 10.1007/s10439-013-0912-5

[47] Bilgen B, Jayasuriya C, Owens B. Current concepts in meniscus tissue engineering and repair. Advanced Healthcare Materials. 2018;**7**(11):1-13. DOI: 10.1002/adhm.201701407

[48] Athanasiou KA, Sanchez-Adams J. In: Athanasiou KA, editor. Engineering the Knee Meniscus. 1st ed. Rice University, USA: Morgan Claypool Publishers; 2009

[49] Van Der Bracht H, Verdonk R, Verbruggen A, Elewaut D, Verdonk P. Cell-based meniscus tissue engineering. In: Ashammakhi N, Reis R, Chiellini E, editors. Topics in Tissue Engineering. Biomaterials and Tissue Engineering Group (BTE); 2007. pp. ch2_1-ch2_13

[50] Scarritt ME, Pashos NC, Bunnell BA. A review of cellularization strategies for tissue engineering of whole organs. Frontiers in Bioengineering and Biotechnology. 2015;**3**(43):1-17. DOI: 10.3389/fbioe.2015.00043

[51] De Bari C, Pitzalis C, Dell'Accio F. Joint tissue engineering. In: Habib NA, Levicar N, Gordon MY, Jiao L, Fisk N, editors. Stem Cell Repair and Regeneration. Vol. 2. London: Imperial College Press; 2007. pp. 107-123

[52] Zuk PA, Zhu M, Ashjian P, De Ugarte DA, Huang JI, Mizuno H, Alfonso ZC, et al. Human adipose tissue is a source of multipotent stem cells. Molecular Biology of the Cell. 2002;**13**:4279-4295

[53] Huang Z, Godkin O, Schulze-Tanzil GG. The challenge in using mesenchymal stromal cells for recellularization of decellularized cartilage. Stem Cell Reviews and Reports. 2016;**13**(1):50-67

[54] Friedenstein AJ, Chailakhyan RK, Latsinik NV, Panasyuk AF, Keiliss-Borok IV. Stromal cells responsible for transferring the microenvironment of the hemopoietic tissues. Cloning in vitro and retransplantation in vivo. Transplantation. 1974;**17**:331-340

[55] Chamberlain G, Fox J, Ashton B, Middleton J. Concise review: Mesenchymal stem cells: Their phenotype, differentiation capacity, immunological features, and potential for homing. Stem Cells. 2007;**25**(11):2739-2749

[56] Yamasaki T, Deie M, Shinomiya R, Izuta Y, Yasunaga Y, Yanada S, Sharman P, Ochi M. Meniscal regeneration using tissue engineering with a scaffold derived from a rat meniscus and mesenchymal stromal cells derived from rat bone marrow. Journal of Biomedical Materials Research. Part A. 2005;**75**(1):23-30

[57] Szilvassy SJ. The biology of hematopoietic stem cells. Archives of

Medical Research. 2003;**34**(6):446-460. DOI: 10.1016/j.arcmed.2003.06.004

[58] Zuk PA, Zhu M, Mizuno H. Multilineage cells from human adipose tissue: Implications for cell-based therapies. Tissue Engineering. 2001;**7**(2):221-228

[59] Moradi L, Vasei M, Dehghan MM, Majidi M, Mohajeri SF, Bonakdar SH. Regeneration of meniscus tissue using adipose mesenchymal stem cells-chondrocytes co-culture on a hybrid scaffold: In vivo study. Biomaterials. 2017;**126**:18-30

[60] De Bari C, Dell'Accio F, Tylzanowski P. Multipotent mesenchymal stem cells from adult human synovial membrane. Arthritis and Rheumatism. 2001;**44**(8):1928-1942

[61] Ozeki N, Muneta T, Matsuta S, Koga H, Nakagawa Y, Mizuno M, et al. Synovial mesenchymal stem cells promote meniscus regeneration augmented by an autologous Achilles tendon graft in a rat partial meniscus defect model. Stem Cells. 2015;**33**(6):1927-1938. DOI: 10.1002/stem.2030

[62] Williams R, Khan IM, Richardson K, Nelson L, McCarthy HE, Analbelsi T, et al. Identification and clonal characterisation of a progenitor cell sub-population in normal human articular cartilage. PLoS One. 2010;**5**(10)

[63] Neumann A, Gardner OF, Williams RA, Alini M, Archer CW, Stoddart MJ, et al. Human articular cartilage progenitor cells are responsive to mechanical stimulation and adenoviral-mediated overexpression of bone-morphogenetic protein 2. PLoS One. 2015;**10**(8):1-17. DOI: 10.1371/journal.pone.0136229

[64] Jayasuriya CT, Owens B, Feltman P, Franco J, Twomey-Kozak J, Newberry J, et al. presented at Orthopaedic Research Society Annual Meeting, New Orleans, LA; March 2018

[65] Zhu WH, Wang YB, Wang L, Qiu GF, Lu LY. Effects of canine myoblasts expressing human cartilage-derived morphogenetic protein-2 on the repair of meniscal fibrocartilage injury. Molecular Medicine Reports. 2014;**9**(5):1767-1772. DOI: 10.3892/mmr.2014.2047

[66] Gu Y, Zhu W, Hao Y, Lu L, Chen Y, Wang Y. Repair of meniscal defect using an induced myoblast-loaded polyglycolic acid mesh in a canine model. Experimental and Therapeutic Medicine. 2012;**3**:293-298

[67] Marsano A, Millward-Sadler SJ, Salter DM, Adesida A, Hardingham T, Tognana E, et al. Differential cartilaginous tissue formation by human synovial membrane, fat pad, meniscus cells and articular chondrocytes. Osteoarthritis and Cartilage. 2007;**15**(1):48-58

[68] Chen YC, Chen RN, Jhan HJ, Liu DZ, Ho HO, Mao Y, Kohn J, Sheu MT. Development and characterization of acellular extracellular matrix scaffolds from porcine menisci for use in cartilage tissue engineering. Tissue Engineering Part C, Methods. 2015;**21**(9):971-986

[69] Wu J, Ding Q, Dutta A, Wang Y, Huang YH, Weng H, Tang L, Hong Y. An injectable extracellular matrix derived hydrogel for meniscus repair and regeneration. Acta Biomaterialia. 2015;**16**:49-59

[70] Peretti GM, Gill TJ, Xu JW, Randolph MA, Morse KR, Zaleske DJ. Cell-based therapy for meniscal repair: A large animal study. The American Journal of Sports Medicine. 2004;**32**:146-158

[71] Hoben GM, Hu JC, James RA, Athanasiou KA. Self-assembly of

fibrochondrocytes and chondrocytes for tissue engineering of the knee meniscus. Tissue Engineering. 2007;**13**(5):939-946

[72] Mauck RL, Martinez-Diaz GJ, Yuan X, Tuan RS. Regional multilineage differentiation potential of meniscal fibrochondrocytes: Implications for meniscus repair. Anatomical Record. 2007;**290**(1):48-58

[73] Niu W, Guo W, Han S, Zhu Y, Liu S, Guo Q. Cell-based strategies for meniscus tissue engineering. Stem Cells International. 2016;**2016**:1-10. DOI: 10.1155/2016/4717184

[74] Fernandes IR, Russo FB, Pignatari GC, Evangelinellis MM, Tavolari S, Muotri AR, et al. Fibroblast sources: Where can we get them? Cytotechnology. 2016;**68**(2):223-228. DOI: 10.1007/s10616-014-9771-7

[75] Stapleton TW, Ingram J, Fisher J, Ingham E. Investigation of the regenerative capacity of an acellular porcine medial meniscus for tissue engineering applications. Tissue Engineering Parts A. 2011;**17**(1-2):231-242